Exercise Balls For Dummies®

Cheat Sheet

An Equipment Checklist

P9-DOG-288

Here's the stuff you definitely need to work out on the ball:

- ✔ An exercise ball (duh).
- ✔ A sticky yoga mat or exercise mat that allows you to kneel or lie on the floor more comfortably. A mat also prevents the ball, your feet, and your hands from slipping and sliding as you perform the exercises.
- ✔ Comfortable workout clothes and sturdy tennis shoes.

Here are some things you may want to buy to enhance your workout:

- ✔ Hand weights
- ✔ Resistance bands
- ✔ Medicine ball
- ✔ Dumbbells

Stuff You Need to Know When Shopping for a Ball

The following is a checklist of questions you should ask and what you need to look for when buying your new ball. Don't forget to tear out this sheet and take it with you!

Ball sizes

The recommended ball size is one that allows you to bend your knees at a 90-degree angle when sitting on the ball with your feet flat on the floor and stacked under your ankles. So, for people

- ✔ Heights 4 feet 8 inches to 5 feet 3 inches, use the 55cm ball.
- ✔ Heights 5 feet 4 inches to 6 feet, use the 65cm ball.
- ✔ Heights over 6 feet, use the 75cm ball.

You may want to use a *larger* ball if you

- ✔ Have longer legs for your height.
- ✔ Are overweight.
- ✔ Have back problems.
- ✔ Are using your ball for a chair or only for stretching.

You may want to use a *smaller* ball if you

- ✔ Have shorter legs.
- ✔ Are at the low end of your height range. For example, if you are 5 feet 4 inches, you may want to use a 55cm ball.

Ball brands

Exercise balls range in price from about $20 to $40, depending on the durability of the ball. I recommend the following brands because they're good quality balls that are made to last.

- ✔ Gymnic fitness ball
- ✔ Duraball
- ✔ Fitball
- ✔ Gymnastik
- ✔ Nautilus

If you find another brand that's cheaper, make sure that it's an anti-bust ball before you buy it.

For Dummies: Bestselling Book Series for Beginners

Exercise Balls For Dummies®

Why Work Out on an Exercise Ball?

You may be wondering what benefits you can expect from working out on the ball. Well, here are just a few:

- Good muscle tone for your entire body
- Improved flexibility
- Better posture for a more graceful appearance
- Stronger core
- Improved cardiovascular system and burning fat with a low-impact workout

Also, you can adapt the ball to your own fitness level, so you don't have to worry about being too out of shape to use it or too in shape to benefit from it.

Top Five Ball Exercises

The following exercises are my personal favorites and are the most effective ones you can do on the ball:

1. Abdominal crunch (see Chapter 8)
2. The bridge (see Chapter 11)
3. Push-up (see Chapter 8)
4. Wall squat (see Chapter 9)
5. Hamstring lift (see Chapter 9)

Relieving Sore Muscles

Starting a workout program or stepping up your current routine often results in some soreness that occurs within 24 hours after your workout. Remember not to overdo it when you're just starting out to prevent an injury. If you start feeling achy or sore (which is different from having a sharp pain immediately after injuring yourself), here are some tips for fast relief:

- If the pain is minor, use ice for the first day or so, and then use heat thereafter.
- If the pain is dull and achy, heat is best to work out the knots.
- If the pain is sharp, use ice to reduce swelling.
- If you're really in pain, try alternating ice and heat for 20 minutes, but always end with ice.

For Dummies: Bestselling Book Series for Beginners

Exercise Balls
FOR
DUMMIES®

by LaReine Chabut

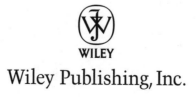

WILEY
Wiley Publishing, Inc.

Exercise Balls For Dummies®

Published by
Wiley Publishing, Inc.
111 River St.
Hoboken, NJ 07030-5774
www.wiley.com

About the Author

LaReine Chabut is an internationally known fitness model, actress, and writer. Certified as a Core trainer with additional certifications in Pilates, personal training, and aerobics, she is the lead instructor for *The Firm*, a popular series of workout videos.

LaReine has graced the covers of such high-profile fitness publications as *Shape, Health, New Body,* and *Runner's World* and has been featured in nationally prominent magazines such as *Allure, People, Newsweek,* and *Glamour.* She has also represented sports giant Nike and swimwear company Body Glove in various print and commercial campaigns. In addition, LaReine has illustrated the rehabilitation guides *The Complete Waterpower Workout Book* (Random House, 1996), *Heal Your Hips* (Wiley, 1999), and *Heal Your Knees* (M. Evans, 2004) and is currently the new face for Nestlé's Good Start Baby Formula.

As a writer, LaReine penned a sitcom pilot entitled "Below the Radar" with Meg Ryan's Prufrock Pictures. She also earned a Clio award nomination for co-writing a public service announcement about Earth Day, which ran in movie theaters nationwide. LaReine has also co-written and starred in two short films: *Separation Anxiety,* which was broadcast on Lifetime Television, and *Good Jill Hunting,* which aired on the Sundance Channel. Her series regular and guest star appearances include *Nash Bridges, The Secret World of Alex Mack, The Single Guy, Linc's, Strange Luck, USA High,* and *Quantum Leap,* to name a few. In films, she has starred opposite Richard Harris and Vincent D'Onofrio.

You can find LaReine's upcoming release, *Lose That Baby Fat!,* in bookstores nationwide in fall 2005.

Dedication

To Bobby and Bella . . . my inspirations. And to all the readers who bought this book because they have a ball and don't know what to do with it. I hope this helps!

Author's Acknowledgments

I would like to acknowledge and warmly thank the following people for helping me along the way (just to name a few): Rob Dyer at Wiley, who encouraged me in the first place to write a book and then quickly gave my name to the acquisitions editor, Natasha Graf. Lynda Huey for referring me to her literary agent and for sharing her wealth of knowledge about the world of fitness. And of course, my literary agent Danielle Egan-Miller and her incredible staff, including Alec MacDonald and Joanna MacKenzie, who endlessly reviewed all my drafts and still correct all my typos.

I also would like to thank the supportive editorial staff at Wiley, starting with Stacy Kennedy, who made me write many sample chapters before I actually got the assignment and helped me become a much faster writer in the process. I also want to thank Chrissy Guthrie, project editor, who added so many fun ideas to the book and made me sound much better than I really do, and copy editor Michelle Dzurny for helping me complete my sentences. I'd also like to thank art coordinator Carmen Krikorian, Melisa Duffy in marketing, and technical editor Kelsey Taylor for their great input and helping make this book a success.

Special thanks to all the models I was fortunate enough to find: Robert Mahl (Chapter 7), Monica Green (technical advisor and Chapters 12, 14, 16, and 17), Karlie Barbato (Chapter 20), Samantha and Pete Johnson (Chapter 20), Tracy Rosenthal (Chapter 18), John Musso (Chapter 19), and Dave Fuhrman (Chapters 8 and 13).

And last but not least, a big thanks goes to photographer Robert Reiff for his beautiful photos, makeup artist Donna Gast, and Nautilus for providing the exercise balls.

Publisher's Acknowledgments

We're proud of this book; please send us your comments through our Dummies online registration form located at www.dummies.com/register/.

Some of the people who helped bring this book to market include the following:

Acquisitions, Editorial, and Media Development

Project Editor: Christina Guthrie

Acquisitions Editor: Stacy Kennedy

Copy Editor: Michelle Dzurny

Editorial Program Assistant: Courtney Allen

Technical Editor: Kelsey Taylor

Senior Permissions Editor: Carmen Krikorian

Editorial Manager: Christine Meloy Beck

Editorial Assistants: Hanna Scott, Nadine Bell, Melissa Bennett

Cover Photo: © Robert Reiff/MagicLight Productions

Cartoons: Rich Tennant (www.the5thwave.com)

Composition Services

Project Coordinator: Adrienne Martinez

Special Art: Interior photos by Robert Reiff/www.magiclight.com

Layout and Graphics: Carl Byers, Andrea Dahl, Joyce Haughey, Clint Lahnen, Barry Offringa, Lynsey Osborn, Amanda Spagnuolo

Proofreaders: Carl William Pierce, TECHBOOKS Production Services

Indexer: TECHBOOKS Production Services

Publishing and Editorial for Consumer Dummies

Diane Graves Steele, Vice President and Publisher, Consumer Dummies

Joyce Pepple, Acquisitions Director, Consumer Dummies

Kristin A. Cocks, Product Development Director, Consumer Dummies

Michael Spring, Vice President and Publisher, Travel

Kelly Regan, Editorial Director, Travel

Publishing for Technology Dummies

Andy Cummings, Vice President and Publisher, Dummies Technology/General User

Composition Services

Gerry Fahey, Vice President of Production Services

Debbie Stailey, Director of Composition Services

Contents at a Glance

Exercises at a Glance

Kid-Friendly Exercises

Lower Body Exercises

Pregnancy-friendly Exercises

Senior-friendly Exercises

Stretches on the Ball

Upper Body Exercises

Warm-up and Cool-down Exercises

Yoga and Pilates Exercises on the Ball

Table of Contents

Introduction

*E*xercise balls, once reserved for only physical therapists and chiropractors, have now entered the mainstream and are on their way to becoming the biggest trend in the fitness world. Using the exercise ball enables you to tighten and tone your abs, improve your core stability, and enhance your balance and coordination like you've never been able to before. Many trends come and go, but using the exercise ball — a simple, inexpensive piece of equipment — in your workout is definitely here to stay.

About This Book

This book introduces you to using the exercise ball in your regular workout routine as well as to a series of specialized ball workouts that include such topics as Pilates, yoga, stretching, and more. You also discover how to stave off workout boredom by adding a few new accessories, such as resistance bands and medicine balls. In addition, I cover weight training, intensive abdominal training, playing around, and simply sitting around.

This book contains comprehensive sections on special circumstances, like staying fit during your pregnancy and keeping your balance throughout seniorhood. I even include a fun-filled ball workout just for kids, which is great for parents to do, too. So whoever you are and whatever your age, you're sure to get a good workout and have a ball while you're doing it!

In this book, I tell you everything you need to know about using an exercise ball. Here's a sampling of some of the questions you can find answers to:

- ✔ How long should a ball workout last?
- ✔ Can everybody use an exercise ball?
- ✔ Are ball classes available?
- ✔ What kind of changes can I expect to see in my body from using the ball?
- ✔ Is it true that mostly physical therapists and chiropractors use the exercise ball?
- ✔ What do I do with my exercise ball?
- ✔ What are the best exercises I can do on the ball?
- ✔ Can kids use the ball to exercise?

✔ Can I use the ball while I'm pregnant?

✔ Is the ball safe for senior citizens?

✔ What if I have back or knee problems? Can I still use the ball?

✔ Will the ball be a challenging enough workout for me if I'm already in shape?

In addition, this book, like all *For Dummies* books, has a friendly and approachable tone that assumes you don't know a whole lot about the subject — not that you're an actual dummy!

Conventions Used in This Book

The focus of this book is on using exercise balls in many different situations while emphasizing safety and proper placement. The ball's round surface makes sitting on the ball relatively difficult, so reading the step-by-step instructions located next to the photo illustrations before you try out any of the actual exercises is important.

Also keep in mind that most exercise illustrations are shown in two stages, labeled A and B, demonstrating a beginning and an end for each pose.

Here are a few additional conventions:

✔ I use *italics* to point out any new terms or bits of jargon you should know.

✔ Web sites and e-mail addresses appear in `monofont` to help them stand out.

✔ The numbered sets of instructions for the exercises and the keywords in lists appear in **boldface.**

What You're Not to Read

Although I feel that all the information in this book is important, the sidebars that appear in the gray boxes don't contain information that you absolutely need to know in order to work out on the ball. However, these sidebars do contain great tips and information about your health, so I encourage you to read them at some point.

Also, any paragraphs marked with the Technical Stuff icon contain interesting but entirely skippable information.

Foolish Assumptions

As I mention earlier in the introduction, this book is for people who don't have a lot of prior knowledge about the subject at hand (in this case, working out using an exercise ball). Keeping this goal in mind, I made a few assumptions about you, the reader:

✔ You're interested in using exercise balls in your fitness program.

✔ You don't have much experience working out on the ball.

✔ You're ready, willing, and able to find out more about the ball and how to actually use it.

If this sounds like you, then you've come to the right place!

How This Book Is Organized

Exercise Balls For Dummies is divided into five different parts, each one with a unique focus. You can go directly to whichever part interests you the most or start at the beginning to gather some information and a checklist of what you need to know before beginning your workout on the ball. Following are the parts and what you can find in them.

Part I: Rolling Exercise Balls into Your Fitness Program

If you're new to using the exercise ball, reading Part I is the way to go. Part I covers all the important issues you want to know *before* you get on the ball.

Part I covers:

✔ *Who* actually created the ball

✔ *What* the ball actually does to provide you with such an amazing workout

✔ *Where* you can purchase the right ball for you

✔ *When* you should use your ball and which situations are the best for using the ball

✔ *Why* you need to know how to sit on the ball properly and how it can lead to a better workout

In Part I, I also offer a chart illustrating your height in relation to the ball (located in Chapter 2), so you're sure to find just the right ball for you.

In addition, Chapter 4 provides photo illustrations that demonstrate the proper alignment of your spine when you're sitting on the ball, which is essential for you to know before you begin working out on the ball.

Part II: Workouts to Have a Ball With

Part II is organized in a very logical manner — Chapter 5 starts off with a series of warm-up exercises on the ball, and then the chapters progress with workouts that are illustrated for various individual body parts. Finally, Chapter 11 finishes with a total body workout.

Because I believe you should work out in a progressive manner (either from the top of the body moving downward or from the bottom of the body and working upward), I strongly encourage starting with the lower-numbered chapters after the warm-up and ending with the cool down in Chapter 10. These chapters concentrate first on the arms, the chest, the abs and back, and the hips and legs.

In Part II, I also cover some of the more intense exercises, such as abdominal crunches and curls in Chapter 8 and some great booty exercises like the wall squat in Chapter 9.

Part III: Variety Is the Spice of Life: Doing Different Activities on the Ball

Part III shows you a variety of different forms of exercise that you can adapt to use on the ball. This section may be the most exciting part of the book for you if you already use another technique, such as yoga or Pilates, and just want to add a few new moves that you can do on the ball. Chapters 12 and 17 illustrate proper breathing for yoga and Pilates along with different poses and exercises that you can do on the ball.

In Chapter 13, I tell you how to weight train by adding heavier dumbbells to your ball workout and by using ankle weights for additional resistance. Chapter 14 (which is my personal favorite) is a chapter on stretching that shows you some really great stretches to do on the ball; this chapter is also a good way to end any of the workouts in this book.

Chapter 15 illustrates a cardio ball workout that not only provides you with a solid workout but also challenges you with a few suggested choreographed ball sequences. Chapter 16 is meant for readers who like to use accessories like resistance bands and a medicine ball to get an even better workout on the ball.

Part IV: Using Exercise Balls in Special Circumstances

Part IV is a dynamic section on special circumstances. If you're pregnant, Chapter 18 is the one for you. This chapter contains some beautiful photo illustrations of a very pregnant model (who gave birth shortly after the photo session) doing a series of stretches and strengthening exercises that help prepare you for that big day.

If you're a senior, Chapter 19 is just for you! It shows the fittest and best-looking 70-year old man I've ever seen doing some amazing hip-strengthening exercises and shoulder stretches that'll help keep you strong and flexible for years to come.

Part IV also contains Chapter 20, a fun-filled chapter for kids and their parents to do together. Or, if that's not possible, you can supervise as your kids bounce, roll, march, side step, and have a ball like our model Karlie did.

Part V: The Part of Tens

In every *For Dummies* book, you find The Part of Tens. The last four chapters in this book contain top-ten lists of fun facts about the different ways that you can use your exercise ball and the different ways that you can complement your ball workout.

In Chapter 24, I give you a list of ten things that you can't do with the ball, which may sound like common sense, but I've found it to be otherwise!

Icons Used in This Book

In this book, you find different pictures in the margins, or *icons,* that give you useful information along the way. Reading these icons before you try the actual exercises is helpful because many of them suggest easier or better ways of performing each one.

Here's a list of icons used in this book:

This icon is for all you hotshots out there who like a good challenge. This icon highlights opportunities to make an exercise more difficult. You find this icon after you've already tried the standard exercise so you can first master it in the beginning stages before you modify it.

As you may have guessed, this icon points out really important information that you need to keep in mind. Very valuable information comes with these icons, so don't skip 'em!

This icon points out info that's good to know, but not necessary to know. If you're in a hurry, you can skip these tidbits.

The Tip icon gives you useful information that'll make your life easier as it relates to exercise balls. I may point you to a specific chapter or resource or provide hints to modify an exercise or to make it easier. For instance, a Tip icon may tell you how to breathe during an exercise to keep you from holding your breath or it may tell you how to stabilize the ball.

The Warning icon highlights information that keeps you from hurting yourself. You should read the information listed under this icon before you attempt the exercise. You'll be glad you did!

Where to Go from Here

Exercise Balls For Dummies is a reference guide for beginners and an introduction to using the ball. You can start reading at the very beginning of this book to gather a little information first or you can dive right in and tear out the yellow Cheat Sheet in the front of this book to take with you as you run out the door to buy your new ball.

If you're not sure where you want to start, I suggest browsing through the table of contents to get a sense of exactly what this book covers and what topics interest you. You may find that you already know the ball basics and have always wanted to try weight training on the ball, so you can immediately flip to that chapter.

If you fall into one of the special circumstances' groups, you may want to go directly to that section to find which chapter covers your special needs. If you're like me, you may just want to go directly to the workout chapters to take a look at the photos and get a sense of how hard you're going to have to work to look like the models.

But seriously, if you know all about the ball already and just want to find out some new exercises or brush up on your skills a bit, you can turn to the index to find out which information pertains to you.

Also be sure to check out www.dummies.com for a list of helpful additional resources. Just type **Exercise Balls** in the search field.

Part I
Rolling Exercise Balls into Your Fitness Program

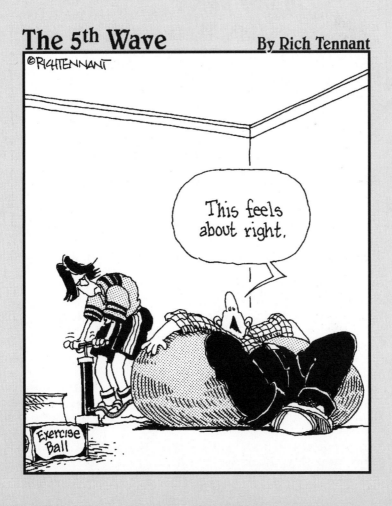

This feels about right.

Exercise Ball

In this part . . .

Part I gives you all the information you need to know to get acquainted with the exercise ball. I cover why the ball is such an amazing fitness tool, who discovered it in the first place, and the principles you need to use the ball. If you've ever wanted to know how to pick the right ball for you or what to wear when you're using it, you can find all that info in this part. I also tell you about all the wonderful benefits your body gets from using the ball — like improving posture, relieving back pain, intensifying your current fitness level, and more! So if you've ever wondered why you should use the ball, this part is for you.

Chapter 1

Having a Ball Getting Fit

*W*hen you go to the gym, do you feel like hurling yourself onto a weight bench? Are you excited to get down on the floor and knock out a few dozen sit-ups? If you answered "no" to these questions, don't worry — you're in good company. In fact, those reasons are why the ball is becoming so popular. The exercise ball is *fun!* And, yes, it does conjure up some really great childhood memories of playing ball in the street or perhaps in your own backyard. So I guess the ball brings out the kid in all of us. And what a great way to approach working out!

In this chapter, you find out who came up with the idea of the exercise ball; what a ball workout can do for you, no matter your fitness level; and how to achieve a healthy lifestyle, both on and off the ball. Finally, at the end of this chapter, you discover two techniques that are the basis for any exercise on the ball — finding neutral spine and setting your abs. Now, let's get the ball rolling!

A Little Background on the Ball

An Italian toymaker named Aquilino Cosani created the *exercise ball* or *stability ball* in 1963. Cosani developed a process for molding the balls out of plastic and then filling them with air and detailing the balls with bright colors. Exercise balls were first sold primarily in Europe to physical therapists and hospitals for rehabilitation under the name Gymnastik. (Later they were called "Swiss balls" because of physical therapist Dr. Susan Klein-Vogelbach's use in Switzerland.) In 1981, Cosani started a new company called Gymnic. These two companies are still in Italy and are the major suppliers of exercise balls throughout the world.

By the late 1980s, physical therapists were using the exercise ball as a rehabilitation tool. In the United States, the first person to put an exercise ball to use was Joanne Posner-Mayer in San Francisco in 1989. Mayer and other physical therapists used the exercise ball for rehabilitating patients with neurological problems. Shortly after, exercise balls crossed over into the world of personal fitness.

Personal trainers began using the ball to enhance their clients' performances; top athletes around the world started using the ball to condition and train their bodies in a new way; and dancers incorporated the ball into their daily regimen to promote better balance and coordination. Before long, exercise balls had jumped into the mainstream in the 1990s. Gyms and workout facilities started offering personal trainers special training courses on the exercise ball and, from there, the ball jumped into the spotlight. With gyms and trainers now offering regular group classes on the ball, the exercise ball is being combined with resistance bands, medicine balls, weights, and other devices to continue making the ball more and more interesting.

The last step for the exercise ball was in-home use. In fact, many people have even replaced their office chairs with a ball. Studies have shown that replacing your chair with the ball increases your focus and concentration, improves your posture, and strengthens your back muscles. If you haven't rolled out your office chair and rolled in the ball, I suggest giving it a try for at least half the time that you sit at your desk.

Who Uses These Balls?

Looking at a simple rubber ball, the exercise ball doesn't seem too intimidating, does it? But these days, everyone from elite athletes to new moms are using the ball to make ordinary exercises more challenging. Traditional exercises, like a simple abdominal crunch, become more effective when you do them on the ball, and the results are twice as fast!

The ball makes a perfect training partner for whatever demographic you happen to fall under. It improves muscle strength and endurance and enhances balance and coordination. By combining the ball with weight training, you can train your core muscles as you pump up your biceps. And you can place the ball under your lower legs to do a few push-ups to get rock hard abs that you wouldn't get just using the resistance of the floor. You can even flatten your post-pregnancy tummy by strengthening your pelvic floor and training your abs, which have been at rest for the last nine months.

Training on the ball really helps members of the following groups improve their level of fitness:

- **Seniors:** Seniors use the ball not only to improve their circulation and posture but also to help stretch and bend, which helps prevent falls.
- **Children:** Children use the ball to improve their focus and coordination while increasing their overall fitness level.
- **Patients:** Patients use the ball to relieve back pain and to strengthen hip and knee joints during post-surgery treatments.
- **Pregnant women:** Mothers-to-be use the ball to stay flexible and comfortable as their tummies grow and to alleviate back pain that the added pressure of carrying around a baby causes.
- **Exercise beginners:** Beginners use the ball to gain stability and balance and to increase flexibility to enhance future training.
- **Athletes:** Athletes use the ball to improve specific skills or sports-specific techniques needed within their individual field of expertise.
- **Yoga students:** Yoga students use the ball as an added base of support while they're moving through postures.
- **Pilates students:** Pilates students use the ball to assist in training their core strength and technique that many of the Pilates exercises emphasize.
- **Birthing moms:** Birthing moms alleviate labor pain by using the ball in different positions to support their body weight.
- **New moms:** New mommies use the ball to tone and strengthen their abdominal muscles after having a baby.
- **Body builders:** Body builders use the ball to alter their base of support and to add resistance.

Why Is the Ball a Great Workout Tool for Me?

Whether you're a serious athlete, a newcomer to exercise, or somewhere in between, reasons abound as to why you should work out on the ball. Besides being inexpensive and portable, exercise balls make working out more fun and interesting, and you can see many other physical benefits after using the ball for just a few weeks.

A ball to have around!

One of the greatest things about owning a ball is that it stares you right in the face as it sits in the corner of your office or your bedroom. Not too easy to avoid it, is it?

Because consistency is the key to exercise, keeping the ball in your house will not only inspire you but it will also help get you going for the long haul. Perhaps you feel like watching television, but you look around and the ball is right next to you. So you roll it out and watch your favorite program as you *sit on it*. Doesn't seem like much, does it? But it is. Just sitting on the ball puts you in touch with your stabilizing muscles and may get you thinking about actually using

them. Otherwise you may just plop down on the couch, and you know you aren't working any muscles that way!

And you can't forget the unavoidable fact that the ball is easy to transport, so you can use the ball wherever you go. Who needs a gym? Simply pump your ball using a hand pump or go to the nearest gas station and use its air pump, and you'll be ready to roll. Even if you take the ball with you and just sit on it to watch one of your favorite in-room movies, you'll be working toward something — consistency. Not too bad for a simple, round, slippery ball, huh?

Here's a list of the most compelling reasons why you should use the exercise ball:

- ✔ The ball provides an *unstable base* (meaning it's difficult to keep still), which makes it an excellent tool for doing challenging exercises that require great strength and control.

- ✔ The ball strengthens your body's core by allowing you to train the deeper abdominal muscles that other pieces of fitness equipment don't reach.

- ✔ You train one muscle group while you use the others for balancing, so the ball helps you tone your entire body.

- ✔ The ball's round shape makes doing back stretches easier and greatly improves your flexibility.

- ✔ Performing abdominal exercises on the ball rather than on the floor significantly increases the tension on your tummy muscles, resulting in a six-pack.

- ✔ As you hold yourself steady on the ball, you get better posture and balance for a more graceful appearance.

- ✔ You can adapt the ball to your own level of fitness simply by keeping the ball closer to your torso, or the core of your body. (As you progress, moving the ball away from your body's core toward your lower legs and feet increases the difficulty.)

✔ Ball exercises use so many of your major muscle groups that your heart rate stays elevated throughout your workout. Ball exercises also improve your cardiovascular system and burn fat with a low-impact workout.

✔ The exercise ball is light and portable, which makes it more convenient than other fitness equipment.

✔ Ball exercises are versatile and easy to modify, so any age group can use them!

Principles of Using the Ball

The principles of using the exercise ball come into play as soon as you combine the instability of the ball (caused by its round shape) with the smooth, hard surface of the floor, which is stable. Just like when practicing Pilates or yoga, you need to follow guidelines to understand how to use the ball. So before you begin your workout, read up on the following principles to gain a better understanding of why the ball is so challenging in the first place.

Proper positioning

You can use quite a few positions with the ball, and they're all dictated by which ball exercises you choose to do. Like with any other piece of equipment, positioning along with proper form is very important.

To make this point a little clearer for you, the following is a list of the most-common ball positions. I also include an example of an exercise that you can do with each position:

✔ **Sitting on the ball:** Abdominal curls (being sure to keep your lower back on the ball as you bend your knees at a 90-degree angle and you rest your feet on the floor)

✔ **Lying backward on the ball:** Backbend stretch (being sure to sit on the ball first and then slowly walk your legs forward until your back is lying backward over the ball)

✔ **Lying sideways on the ball:** Lateral curls or side stretch (being sure to first kneel on the floor and position your right hip and side against the ball)

✔ **Lying forward on the ball or on your tummy:** The drape, or draping your body over the ball (being sure to place your feet on the floor behind you and your hands on the floor in front of you)

✔ **Lying on the floor with your legs on the ball:** Hamstring lifts or roll away (being sure to press your lower legs into the ball and rest your arms by your sides on the floor)

Range of motion

Because the ball moves freely, it creates a wider range of motion for working your joints and keeping them flexible as opposed to working with a weight bench. When you train on the ball, you use a full range of motion and recruit additional muscle groups to maintain proper form.

The ball's full range of motion serves as a kind of *check and balance system* because, if you don't do each exercise correctly, you fall on your butt! Keeping the ball steady lets you know immediately whether or not you're maintaining good posture and proper form.

Coordination and balance

When you take away the stability of a chair and sit on the ball, you change your center of gravity and alter the way you need to sit; that is, you sit up straight (otherwise known as having good posture).

Working on coordination and balance at the same time recruits the brain and the muscles, so you get more bang for your buck while working out on the ball. Using your *stabilizing muscles* (deeper abdominal muscles) to maintain your balance and concentrating so you don't fall off the ball may be the two most important principles of working with the ball.

Reaping the Benefits

Besides developing good overall muscle tone for your entire body, the ball provides numerous other benefits that range anywhere from rehabilitating back, hip, and knee injuries to delivering a powerful workout to improve core stability, posture, and muscle balance. You also improve your flexibility and your cardiovascular system by using a low-impact workout.

Following are a few of the most important benefits for anyone wanting to use the ball and get a little background on what exactly you're supposed to be working. Additionally, you can find a list of the benefits of using the ball during pregnancy in Chapter 18, and I cover the benefits of working out on the ball for seniors in Chapter 19.

Back and spine health

The ball is great if you have back problems because it supports your lower back as you exercise and stretch. And that's exactly why physical therapists and chiropractors started using the ball for therapy. So many people suffer from back strain and injuries these days that thinking of anyone you know who hasn't is a challenge. Take my uncle, for example, who recently came home from the chiropractor's office with a ball (which I was sure would sit in the corner and collect dust) but, to my surprise, he uses it every day! What other object can you think of that you can simply lay your body over and feel instant relief? Not too many.

You can find many simple stretches in Chapter 14 and other chapters that provide not only back stretches but also a series of strengthening exercises for your entire back.

Killer abs

You can expect to get strong abs from training on the ball. And, as you may already know, strong abs means a strong, healthy back to help support all your movements throughout the day. In fact, studies have shown that people like to work their abs more than any other body part.

So why is the ball so great for giving you killer abs and strengthening your back? Well, that question has two very good answers:

✔ When you lie with your back on the floor to do a sit-up, you're using a stable base to support your back. This flattened-out position results in moving and training your abdominal muscles in only one direction: upward as you lift your shoulders off the floor and bring your elbows to your knees.

✔ When you do abdominal exercises on the ball, you increase the level of resistance because your spine curves naturally around the ball when you lift up to do a crunch, plus you're able to use a full range of motion rather than the limited one you get when you use the floor. Simply put, because of the ball's round shape, you get a lot more range of motion in your spine than you do using the flatness of the floor.

Doing abdominal exercises on the ball is more challenging in other ways, too. Because you need to incorporate other muscle groups to help you keep your balance on the ball, you use more muscles and strengthen more than just your tummy area:

✔ You use your glutes when you squeeze them together and contract as you lift up toward the ceiling.

✔ Your hamstrings contract as you press down into the floor to keep the ball steady.

✔ Your hip flexors tighten and release as you bend at the waist into the curled-up position of an abdominal crunch.

As an end result of training on the ball, you can expect to see improved posture, increased balance, and increased strength in your back muscles. Now that's what I call amazing!

Core stability

With so much talk these days about working your "core," you may be wondering what the heck your core actually is. Well, the core is the muscles in your body that stabilize and support all your movements. Your core, or what people used to call your "midsection," is made up of the deep abdominal and back muscles that work as stabilizers for your entire body. These muscles are the "deep" muscles because, although you cannot see them, they maintain the core stability in your body.

The three muscles in the midsection, or "trunk" of your body, are

- *Transverse abdominus:* The deep abdominal muscles
- *Tultifidus:* The back muscles that support the lumbar spine
- *Quadratus lumborum:* The muscles of the lower back that maintain spinal and pelvic balance

These muscles work together to protect your spine and help with everyday activities. Lifting, throwing, bending, reaching, and running use the stabilizer muscles, so keeping them well-conditioned is extremely important. Without conditioned stabilizer muscles, simple movements like pulling, walking, and running go unsupported and leave you at risk for injuries.

Training on the ball is one way to work this group of hard-to-reach muscles. Just by sitting on the ball, you're able to activate the stabilizer muscles and not only improve your posture, but you also feel more in touch with your center of gravity. This is just one of the many benefits you get from adding exercise balls to your fitness program.

The additional core muscles that lie deep within your body and are impossible to see from the outside include the pelvic floor and are otherwise described as the muscles that run from your tailbone to your pubic bone. (I like to refer to the pelvic floor as the "girdle" muscles because they keep everything sucked in!)

To tighten the pelvic floor, you simply activate the muscles you use when you're desperately looking for a bathroom and can't find one! (Your muscles should feel as if you're trying to "hold it" or keep from going to the bathroom.) Just sitting on the ball activates these muscles. At first, keeping your balance may be difficult because the ball is an unstable base and requires you to have great strength in your back and abdominal muscles.

When you sit on a chair or a weight bench at the gym, you certainly don't use any of these stabilizing muscles that your body calls upon while you're working out on the ball. By bringing your feet closer together when you're sitting on the ball, you can intensify your workout by altering your base of support. After a few sessions on the ball, you will become more aware and be able to identify how your core should feel when you're engaging it and will soon be able to maintain your balance on the ball just as you would if you were sitting on a chair.

For training your core on the ball, the rule of thumb is: The farther away the ball is from the core of your body, the more difficult maintaining your balance is. For example, when doing a push-up on the ball, placing the ball underneath your lower legs makes doing the push-up much easier because the ball is closer to your core. To increase the difficulty, all you have to do is roll the ball out to your feet so it's farther away from the center of your body, and so maintaining your balance is harder.

Posture

Being a dancer for many years in New York, I was always told to press my back "into" the floor or to have a "flat" back. Nowadays, experts have found that maintaining the slight natural curve in your spine is healthier. When using the ball, maintaining this natural curve is important to help you keep from arching your back and to protect the spine.

Chapter 4 shows photo illustrations of the three different kinds of postures you can use when sitting on the ball. The best of the three is called *neutral spine.* I describe the benefits of maintaining a neutral spine in this chapter and throughout this book.

Muscle balance

When one muscle group is stronger than its opposing muscle group, this causes a *muscle imbalance.* Muscles that need to work together to perform a particular task, such as the triceps and biceps, are a good example of muscle groups that can have a muscle imbalance.

The muscles that are in the front of your body, or the *anterior muscles,* are naturally stronger than the muscles that lie along the back of your body, otherwise known as the *posterior muscles,* because you use them more frequently throughout the day. To complicate the matter further, most people tend to over-train their anterior muscles and neglect their posterior muscles, which can create bad posture and additional imbalances.

The ball offers a solution to muscle imbalances because it supports the lower back and other posterior muscles during training. To look and feel good, whether you're coming or going, you need to train your buttocks, back, and hamstrings. And maybe concentrate a little less on those biceps!

Beyond the Ball: Being Fit for Life?

With so many diet products, fitness gimmicks, sports drinks, and magic pills on the market today, knowing what really works and what you really need to do to get and stay healthy is tough.

Although you've heard or read it all before, the answer is really pretty simple: You need to dedicate yourself and have lots of patience. Here are a few more things you can do that will definitely do the trick.

Eating a healthy diet

Some people think that if they exercise, they don't have to watch what they eat. Although exercise does give you more leeway, you still need to be mindful of the quality and quantity of food you eat each day because your body has to burn off what you eat through your daily activities. Portion control or cutting calories works best for just about everybody.

Try eating five or six times a day to stave off hunger and to keep you going all day long. Eating on this schedule is better than waiting all day to eat one huge meal at night when you have no time left to burn off all those calories!

To keep your energy up and your blood sugar from dipping (plus boost your metabolism), each small meal should be around 300 to 500 calories, which translates into an apple, a yogurt, and a slice of cheese.

Knowing what a balanced diet includes these days is tough, especially if you've ever taken a look at the Food Guide Pyramid. If you read that guide, you'll be eating six to eleven servings of bread, rice, pasta, and cereal. Yikes! A good balanced diet consists of some form of protein (lean meats, fish, and tofu), veggies, fruits, dairy, and *good* carbs (see the list of good carbs in the sidebar "My take on the low-carb craze"). In addition, staying away from white sugar and white flour and steering toward whole grains and whole oats should help you on your way to eating healthier in no time.

Having an effective workout program

To avoid heart disease and other chronic illnesses, you have to fit in some form of exercise to get your circulation flowing and your heart pumping. You'll also see and feel a difference in your energy level in no time after you try one of the following suggested workouts.

✔ **Aerobic exercise:** Try to spend at least 20 to 60 minutes three to five days a week doing some form of aerobic exercise. Activities such as walking, hiking, biking, jogging, cross-country skiing, and skating are great ways to get in shape. But make sure you choose an exercise that you enjoy and can easily include in your schedule.

✔ **Strength training:** Depending on your individual fitness level, strength-training sessions should start at 30 minutes and increase to 60 minutes as you feel the need for more intensity and a higher weight. Be sure to take a look at the weight-training chapter (Chapter 13) and the shapely arms chapter (Chapter 7), which offer a variety of strength-training exercises on the ball.

✔ **Flexibility training:** You should do flexibility and stretching exercises at least 20 minutes a day or three times a week in an hourly session. To increase your flexibility, try the exercises in Chapter 12 (doing Pilates on the ball) or Chapter 17 (doing yoga on the ball). To get a good stretch, try the exercises in Chapter 14 (a stretching workout on the ball).

My take on the low-carb craze

I couldn't get away without discussing the war on carbs (carbohydrates) somewhere in this book. Well, this info may come as a surprise to some of you, but all carbs are not bad! Indeed, some carbs are good, and keeping them in your diet is important so your body doesn't lose the precious muscle that's responsible for burning up a great deal of your daily calories. And we all know that quick-fix diets (like no-carb diets) are hard to maintain and, in the long run, end up backfiring, right?

Just as skipping meals all day only leads to failure (you eat like an animal when nighttime comes), so does trying to eat only bacon and sausage all day. The idea may sound good to you right now but, after a few weeks of stuffing your face with only protein, believe me, you'll be craving some fresh fruit. So here are a few hints on good carbs and bad carbs; and remember, like anything in life, moderation is the key:

✔ **The good carbs:** Fresh fruits, *whole grain* breads and cereals, vegetables, oatmeal, beans, potatoes, or anything that's not processed and contains some small amount of fiber.

✔ **The bad carbs:** Sugar, starches made from *white* flour (cookies and cakes), white bread, white rice, white pasta, soda, and any sugary food, such as ice cream. Basically, anything that's processed or refined is a bad carb.

Some really good snack choices are still available when you're watching your carb intake. A few of these are dried fruit, fresh fruits, cheese crackers, peanut butter crackers, trail mix, yogurt, vanilla wafers, grain crackers, and granola bars. Also, many companies offer low-carb alternatives (which means they make their foods without *white* sugar and *white* flour).

People who are on a low-carb diet should increase their fiber intake and drink plenty of water to keep their bodies hydrated and to replace the lost fiber that comes from incorporating many forms of carbohydrates in your diet.

Don't forget cross training

A workout can get boring when you've done it for a while. So give yourself a pat on the back for mastering it, but move on to something else — quickly. Unfortunately, when people get bored with their workout, they may get discouraged with working out altogether. *Cross training*, or doing a variety of workouts, not only gives you something new to master, but it also changes your body almost overnight. For example, if you're a swimmer and feel that you're over-training the muscles in your upper body, taking a step aerobics class not only can add variety to your fitness routine, but it will work and build the muscles in your lower body and legs, leaving you looking shapelier and stronger in no time. Now that's exciting!

Cross training is essential to any exercise program because it keeps you from getting tired of one particular workout. If you're a runner and are used to running everyday, the muscles in your body will eventually reach a plateau and you'll stop seeing improvement in your level of fitness.

Here are a few suggestions for keeping things fresh and staying in tip-top shape:

✔ If you're into cardio, try working your upper body by lifting weights or using resistance bands to strengthen and tone the muscles that don't get an intense workout while you're running or walking.

✔ If you're into lifting weights, you may want to try taking a yoga or Pilates class to stretch out the muscles and increase your flexibility.

Avoiding boredom and keeping your fitness regimen new and challenging will provide your body with changes that may surprise even you.

In addition, make sure that each workout includes an ample warm-up and a cool down. See Chapters 5 and 10 for ways to warm up and cool down using the ball.

Most importantly, listen to your body. Slow down or rest when you feel out of breath or uncomfortable. Increasing your exercise time and intensity too quickly sets you up for injury.

Setting realistic goals

Being motivated to start something new is great, but buying all the equipment you need for a new sport and then not using it or joining a new gym and never using your membership isn't. Slow and steady wins the race. Keep your ultimate goal in mind as you begin something new and have the patience and determination to see it through. You'll see the results sooner rather than later. Some good guidelines for a beginner are

Got 10 minutes?

You can find so many excuses to use to keep from working out. But probably the number-one excuse is that you don't have the time! Well, that old excuse is null and void in the world of health and fitness, because the latest trend in getting your daily cardio and toning up is by doing ten-minute workouts twice daily or even once daily, if that's all you have time for.

Many a man or woman felt defeated, thinking he or she needed a whole hour or an uninterrupted segment of time to get in a good workout. The solution? *Hi-Lo Cardio.* Anyone and everyone who has ten minutes can greatly benefit from these broken down training intervals, even if you have to do them over your lunch hour, while your baby naps, instead of taking a shower (only

new moms are excused), or before you head out the door to start your day.

Try doing any cardiovascular activity (say the treadmill) for three minutes at a low intensity to warm up your body; then switch to a moderate intensity for two minutes; follow it with two minutes of the highest intensity you can handle; then slow your intensity for the last three minutes. This workout boosts your metabolism and spikes your heart rate into the fat-burning zone. And all in ten minutes! Doing cardio ball exercises (see Chapter 15), jumping rope, doing the elliptical trainer, running up and down stairs, spinning on a bike, and doing jumping jacks all do the trick.

✔ **Pick something that you can easily fit into your schedule and use consistently.** The recommended workout time for someone just getting started is two to three times a week for 30 minutes or longer. As you build your endurance and level of fitness, you should gradually increase your level of intensity to three or four times a week for 30 minutes or longer.

✔ **Avoid over-training.** When you first begin exercising, never let yourself get fatigued to the point that you can't hold a conversation or are short of breath.

A good starting point is to buy an exercise ball (because they're inexpensive and a lot of fun). Use it right away by replacing your desk chair for at least one hour a day while you're working at your computer. You'll notice a difference right away because when you're using the ball as a chair, you're forced to sit up straight with both feet on the floor to remain steady and to engage your stabilizing muscles. At the end of the day, you'll feel you did something better for yourself than just sitting around.

Get Ready, Get Set . . .

To get familiar with the ball, first you have to develop an awareness of how you're sitting and what you need to do to stay seated on it. The following exercises help you get acquainted with the proper alignment (neutral spine) that you need to use and help you set your abs, which you need to do before you perform each exercise. Both these exercises are fun and important activities to master before you begin your workout. After you master finding neutral spine and setting your abs, you'll be ready for anything on the ball!

Finding neutral spine

When your car is in neutral, you know that it's in a "pause" mode, but does neutral mean the same thing in physiology? You often hear the term "neutral spine" used in exercise, but what is it really?

Being in neutral spine is really an active position where you engage your lower abdominal and pelvic stabilizer muscles to create a "girdle" to enable your body to protect itself from injury.

To keep your back from arching and to practice neutral spine, try this exercise in front of a mirror:

1. **Stand facing the side as you look into a mirror.**

2. **Imagine a ruler extending along your back from the top of your shoulders or shoulder blades to the bottom of your pelvis or hips.**

3. **Stand tall and straight so everything stacks up neatly as follows: head, shoulders, rib cage, pelvis, and legs.**

You can also try this exercise by lying with your back on the floor:

1. **Lie on the floor with your back pressed down. If your back is flat, you shouldn't be able to put your hand between the floor and your back.**

2. **As you exhale, bring your knees to your chest and think about the placement of your back on the floor.**

3. **Hold your knees into your chest for a few moments, and then release your legs back to the floor.**

Notice how your back feels now. Is it pressed down and not arching? Can you feel the neutral position of your body as it relaxes on the floor but is still actively pressing downward? This position is called *neutral spine* and is the proper alignment that you use with all exercise ball programs.

Setting your abs

Working out on the ball is different than sitting in a chair because the ball is round and has an uneven surface. At first, these differences may not seem like a big deal to you but, in reality, it is! You need time and practice to have control and master some, if not all, the exercises in this book.

To do the workouts in this book, you need to know how to tighten your abdominal muscles while keeping your spine long and straight. This position is called "setting your abs." Setting your abs allows you to develop strength throughout your core muscles and helps you develop an awareness of where your movements originate.

The following is a list of the steps you should take each time you get on the ball to set your abs:

1. **Sit tall on the ball with your feet hip-distance apart and firmly planted on the ground.**

2. **Take a deep breath and visualize a belt tightening around your waist.**

3. **Let your rib cage lift and fill with air.**

4. **Place one hand below your belly button and feel the tightening and lifting.**

5. **Place your other hand on the small of your back to feel the natural curve of your spine as you're sitting tall on the ball.**

6. **As you exhale, keep your hand on your lower abdominal muscles or below your belly button to make sure the tightening remains.**

When you set your abs properly, you should feel that you're ready for anything, as if someone were going to punch you in the stomach and you were bracing yourself for the punch.

After a while, setting your abs will become almost second nature to you. You'll be able to see the difference in your posture immediately and in how you move throughout your day.

You never want to hold your breath when you're working out on the ball because as soon as you let it out, you may lose your balance.

Chapter 2

Choosing the Right Ball for *You*

. . . .

In This Chapter

▶ Finding the right size ball for you

▶ Considering special circumstances

▶ Evaluating a ball's quality

▶ Deciding where to buy your new ball

▶ Finding out what it costs to purchase a ball

▶ Adding heavy balls and accessories to your shopping list

. . . .

A ball's a ball, right? Well, yes and no. Exercise balls may all look the same, but all exercise balls are *not* created equally. Fitness trends may come and go, but just as physical therapists and chiropractors have discovered, the exercise ball is here to stay. And wouldn't buying one that'll be around as long as you are be nice?

In this chapter, you discover how to choose your new ball based on three important factors: size, level of comfort, and quality. Because exercise balls can vary greatly from manufacturer to manufacturer, knowing the answers to these questions, among others like "Which balls are anti-burst?" and "Which ball is the right height for you?" is important. When you choose a new ball, you should do it with confidence and the knowledge that you're getting the most for your money.

Another bonus feature of this book is the Cheat Sheet (the little yellow card located in the very front), which you can tear out and take with you when you go to purchase your new ball. The Cheat Sheet lists the most important criteria for purchasing a ball. Be sure to take a look at the accessories that you really should consider when purchasing your new ball (see Chapter 16). Medicine balls, heavy balls, and resistance bands are great ways to add variety to your workout, and you often find them in the same aisles or on the same Web sites as exercise balls.

Exercise Balls
Right Fit

...you use the ball with so many different body positions while you're ...rcising, the size of the ball you use really does make a difference and can make or break your workout.

To give you an example of this fact, I was recently in a ball class at the gym. By the time I arrived, all the balls for my height had been taken. Naturally, I took the next size up, thinking that I could make it work, but I had a really difficult time finishing the class. In the first place, many of the exercises required sitting on the floor with the ball positioned between my legs. Using a larger ball than you need makes seeing over the ball extremely difficult (if not impossible) when you're in that position. Next, I had to position the ball between my knees and roll onto my back. Sounds easy enough, but because the ball was too large, it pressed my legs down toward the floor and my hips started to hurt! Ouch! (I've been through childbirth, and I don't feel like repeating that feeling in a ball class.)

The point is, size does matter. And although using smaller balls can enhance certain exercises and larger balls can support your body weight if you have a bad back, using the right ball for *you,* which means one that is measured by your height and/or your arm span, makes all the difference in the world.

Using your height to size up your ball

When you stand next to an exercise ball, it should be even or slightly above your knee level. The best way to size up your ball is by sitting on it. When you sit on the ball, your knees should be bent at a 90-degree angle and your thighs should be parallel or even with the floor. Figure 2-1 provides a quick illustration. Find your height and see which ball size you should try first.

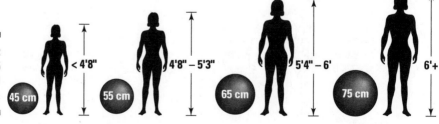

Figure 2-1: 45 cm to 75 cm ball and height chart.

The following chart shows a slight variation of recommended heights for the different ball sizes you can choose from.

Height	Recommended ball size
Under 4'8"	45 cm ball
4'8" to 5'3"	55 cm ball
5'4" to 6'	65 cm ball
6' and over	75 cm ball

For kids who are 5 years and younger, always use a 45 cm ball.

Doing the sit test

The best way to tell whether or not your new ball is the correct height is to sit on it. The recommended height allows you to bend your knees at a 90-degree angle when you're sitting on the ball and your feet are flat on the floor. This angle allows your hips to be level or slightly higher than your knees.

A ball that's too small compromises the position of your hips and pelvis when you sit on it, whereas a ball that's too large doesn't allow your feet to touch the ground, making it unstable. Achieving a good balance between a ball that's too large or a ball that's too small provides you with the best work-out. As Goldilocks once said, not too hard, not too soft, juuuuussssst right.

Lying on the ball

When you lie on your stomach on the ball, you want to make sure that your back doesn't arch. Your back should maintain the natural curve, otherwise known as *neutral spine*. If you arch your back at all when you lie face down with your stomach on ball, you need to get a smaller ball so you avoid injury from placing strain on your back. In addition, when you lie face down on the ball, your hands should be able to comfortably touch the floor in front of you.

Using your arm to size up your ball

Another way to find the correct size ball is to measure the length of your arm from your fingertip to your shoulder. Because people have different leg lengths (some have shorter legs and some have longer legs), using your arm span to find a ball that's just right for you can be a more accurate way to measure a ball. If you plan to use the ball for a lot of aerobic exercise and need to hold onto it, using your arm measurement can provide a better fit for your circumstances. However, using your arm-span measurement to buy your new ball can take a bit more time and a bit more skill because most people are more familiar with their height rather than their arm span. If you choose to use this method of measuring, take a look at the following chart to see where you fit in.

Arm length	Recommended ball size
22" to 25½"	55 cm ball
26" to 31½"	65 cm ball
31¾" to 35½"	75 cm ball

Beyond Height: Special Circumstances That Can Affect Your Choice

To make sure you get just the right ball for you, know the answers to the following questions before you go out and purchase your ball.

✔ Do you have long or short legs?

✔ Are you a beginning exerciser or an advanced exerciser (you work out five or more times per week)?

✔ Do you have knee problems of any kind?

✔ Do you have back problems?

✔ Are you overweight?

✔ Do you plan to use the ball only for stretching?

After you've answered these questions, read on to find out which ball is the perfect fit for you.

Longer or shorter legs

If you're lucky and have long legs (and you know who you are), you may want to use a larger ball because it allows your knees to remain parallel to the floor. Keeping your knees parallel to the floor not only makes the exercises more effective, but it also keeps your pelvis on the same plane or in line with your hips and knees, enabling you to engage your stabilizing muscles.

On the other hand, if you have shorter legs or are at the end of your height range, you may want to use a smaller ball because, if you can't plant your feet firmly on the ground, you won't be able to keep the ball steady. So, for example, say you're 5 feet 4 inches; you may want to use a 55 cm ball rather than a 65 cm ball.

Color is personal

Although the fitness industry doesn't really have standard colors for identifying ball sizes, manufacturers may have some method to their madness when they choose colors for the general public. If you've never had your colors analyzed before, here's your chance. Just check out the chart of colors to see if you're a gray, purple, green, red, blue, or yellow personality.

If you pick the color gray: You're content and like to play it safe. Some may say that you have neutral feelings about things, but you really just like to protect yourself. You're the opposite of anyone who would choose the color red, because you don't need or want the attention and are willing to work hard for everything in life.

If you picked the color purple: You're intriguing and have an aura of mystery about you. You're very spiritual and highly creative, which most likely means that you're an artist or in some form of the arts. Those who feel they're unconventional like the color purple. Purple people are very giving and can sometimes be quite charming — but not all the time! Very smart and super sensitive, you posses conflicting traits just like the two colors that make up the color purple — red and blue (red being the thrill-seeker, and blue being the balanced nature-lover). You may be easy to get along with but, in the end, you're really hard to get to know.

If you picked the color green: You're balanced and stable because green is nature's most abundant and beautiful color, which represents warmth and coolness. You're an involved parent and are a good neighbor, patriotic, and active in all that concerns you. Plus, you're a neat freak (no wonder I picked a green ball) who's generous, kind, and likes to do things for others. You're also extremely sensitive to doing just the right thing.

If you picked the color red: You're impulsive, active, intense, and competitive (not to mention aggressive and passionate). The color red is only for people who are exciting, optimistic, emotional, and extroverted. You desire to live and love and truly experience life to its fullest. From a physiological standpoint, red can speed up your pulse, increase your rate of breathing, and raise your blood pressure. So if you choose red, you want to be noticed. Exciting!

If you picked the color blue: You're in good company, because blue is the most popular color in the world today. It represents peace and tranquility. Blue is the color of harmony, so you're even-tempered and reliable. You're patient and show strong perseverance in the face of adversity; "slow and steady wins the race" is your motto. Although you have a tendency to be a perfectionist (maybe I should have a blue ball), your gentle nature keeps you from being overly harsh on those around you.

If you picked the color yellow: You're warm and love the sunshine. You're very active and are definitely an upbeat person. You're very imaginative and creative and you're also ambitious and often achieve success as a result of your great outlook on life. You crave challenges and tend to be a perfectionist. Although you're a winner and don't like being second-best, you're a good sport and a good friend.

To make your workout more dynamic, choose one of these fun colors for your new exercise ball. Just make sure the color fits your personality and the décor of your home because your new ball will most likely be hanging around your house when you're not using it (probably in the corner somewhere).

Your level of fitness

If you aren't really athletic, are new to working out, or are beginning a new fitness program, using a larger ball is probably best for you because it's easier to control and provides a more stable base. Kind of like when you're beginning to surf and need to use a long board until you get the hang of it and can switch to a short board.

I recommend working up slowly (or maybe that's working down) to a smaller ball. After you've gained more control and balance, using a smaller ball will be easier and will come more naturally to you.

Knee problems

I have a book that just came out called *Heal Your Knees* (M. Evans). In this book, I illustrate a land and pool program for rehabilitating knee injuries (even the photographer who shot the beautiful photographs for this book had to have knee surgery in between photo shoots!). Knee problems are way too common these days, and using the ball is a great way to rehabilitate them. And I'll tell you why.

The ball is a great way to rehabilitate knee injuries because it doesn't place strain on the knee joint if you make sure your knees are bent at a 90-degree angle when you're sitting on the ball. However, using a ball that is too small puts more strain on your knees than a larger ball because of the slight downward sloping position. Therefore, I recommend using a larger ball for anyone who has undergone knee surgery or experiences pain in their knee joints during exercise.

Back problems

Physical therapists first used the ball to help treat back injuries because it provides a unique base for supporting the lower back. So if you or someone you know has back problems, don't feel uneasy about working out with the ball — you're a prime candidate!

If you've had back surgery or back pain, I recommend getting a larger ball because it lifts and supports your body's weight by not allowing your hips to sink lower than your back. Using a larger ball allows your hips and lower back to exist on the same plane, allowing your thighs to remain parallel to the floor, which prevents injury and strain on your lower back.

Being overweight

If you're carrying around extra body weight, I recommend using a larger ball because you can slightly under-inflate it. Under-inflating your ball allows you to adjust its height according to your weight. When you need to under-inflate a ball, make sure that your thighs are parallel to the floor and your feet remain flat on the ground. If you find yourself sinking too far into the ball, you can add more air to adjust it accordingly.

The 75 cm ball or the largest exercise balls are tested to hold more than 600 pounds, with the combined weight of your body and weights that you use as accessories. If you're anywhere near this weight, use the largest ball to be sure that you have the best base of support that's available to you (look for the *firm ball,* listed as one of the accessories in this chapter under "For those who love gadgets and gizmos: Great new accessories" later in this chapter).

A ball for stretching

For stretching, use a larger ball because you can drape your body more comfortably over the ball. A larger ball also allows the natural force of gravity to assist you while you're performing many of the stretching positions or poses in this book.

In fact, a new ball called a *stretching ball* is out on the market and it's for stretching only. This ball is 75 cm, which is larger than you need for aerobics or strength training. To find out about a stretching ball and why it's gaining popularity, flip to Chapter 14.

Strength training

If you plan to use the ball primarily for strength training (like in Chapter 7 or Chapter 13), I recommend using a smaller ball. Using a smaller ball gives you a greater range of motion than a larger ball does for the pulling, pushing, and lifting you need to do with hand weights or dumbbells.

In addition, a smaller ball offers a shorter base, which allows you to be closer to the ground so you can pick your weights and your water bottle up off the floor more easily.

Considering Different Qualities of Balls

So many different types and qualities of balls are available on the market today. Some are good, and some are not so good. Here's the rule of thumb for distinguishing a good ball from a bad one: Steer away from balls that are super shiny or slippery because they're usually made from a material that deteriorates easily.

The following is a list of ball guidelines for you to look for when you're purchasing a ball:

- **Burst-resistant or anti-burst:** The most widely used balls are burst-resistant and are used by physical therapists and personal trainers. These balls are stronger than others and maintain their shape for longer periods of time.

- **Perfectly round:** This point may seem obvious, but make sure your new ball is perfectly round. Inexpensive balls can actually lose their shape because they lose air over a short period of time, and you need to refill them to maintain their roundness. A good quality ball should maintain its round shape until it's noticeably smaller or has more give to it than when you started using it.

- **Weight-tested:** Balls should be weight-tested to more than 600 pounds, including accessories.

- **Latex-free material:** A ball made out of vinyl or a latex-free material is best for firmness. In addition, a latex-free material won't be slippery, so you can maintain control of the exercises and your movements better. You also need a soft rubber ball to cushion and support your weight, so the material your ball is made out of is very important.

- **Designed to deflate slowly if punctured:** Unless you want your ball to pop like a balloon, look for one that deflates slowly in case you roll over a tack or puncture it.

What to Pay for Your New Ball

Most balls range in price from $20 to $40, depending on the material and the manufacturer. The size of the ball affects the price slightly but not too much. For example, the smaller balls (45 cm) are usually around $20, whereas the larger balls (75 cm) usually cost around $30. In addition, if the ball is made of an anti-burst material and has been weight-tested up to 1,000 pounds, you can expect to pay in the higher range.

As with any type of purchase, you get what you pay for. So if you pay a little more for a well-known brand, it will cost you more now but, in the end, will last longer and be more durable.

Where to Purchase Your New Ball

Although discount superstores and many other retail stores carry exercise balls, the exercise ball is mass-produced in Europe (because the first exercise ball was invented by Italian toymaker Aquilino Cosani in Italy). In fact, the largest direct source of Italian-manufactured balls in the United States is Fitball. These balls are of the highest quality, and I find them to be more durable than other types. The following is a list of locations where you can purchase these well-made European brands of balls.

Retail store locations

You can find Gymnic fitness balls, Duraballs, Fitballs, and Gymnastik at the stores and locations listed here.

Here's a list of distributors in the United States:

- ✔ The Gym Ball Store
- ✔ Relax The Back Stores
- ✔ The Comfort Store
- ✔ ERGO-I-AM
- ✔ Orthopedic Physical Therapy Products (ORTO)
- ✔ Bheka Yoga Supplies
- ✔ The Saunders Group
- ✔ Grateful Back

The following is a list of distributors in Canada:

- ✔ IncrediBall

The following is a list of distributors in Mexico:

- ✔ PRO-GYM

Internet sites

Isn't the Internet great for purchasing stuff? Now you can go online and get practically anything that you're looking for without fighting traffic! Ah, modern conveniences.

If you're the type of person who doesn't need to actually see what you're buying first (other than a picture like most Web sites display), then shopping on the Internet is for you. Ball Dynamics is the leading distributor of exercise balls, so if you go to the company's Web site, you can locate many of the brands I mention earlier in this chapter or try one of the direct manufacturer Web sites that I list here.

Most companies provide a money-back guarantee if you're not completely satisfied, so what do you have to lose?

- ✔ www.balldynamics.com
- ✔ www.gymball.com
- ✔ www.fitball.com
- ✔ www.bodytrends.com
- ✔ www.spriproducts.com
- ✔ www.fitter1.com
- ✔ www.resistaball.com

Sporting goods stores

Sporting goods stores are great for buying balls these days. But you don't see too many balls on display at the store because they're packaged in boxes. Even so, most brands of balls sold at sporting goods stores are packaged as a kit containing videos or wall charts providing demonstrations of actual ball exercises. Most of these kits also contain hand pumps or foot pumps so you can fill your ball with air when you get home and are ready to go (see Chapter 3 for a better, faster way to inflate your ball).

The gym

When you walk onto the training floor at your local gym or health center, you'll notice an abundance of balls these days. (Many gyms provide group classes for the public and already provide a ball for you.)

Gyms that carry balls usually sell them at the retail stores located inside the clubs. At the club retail stores, most balls are already filled with air, which serves two purposes:

✔ You can see the actual size of the ball and try it out.

✔ Professionals can fill the ball with air to its correct diameter.

Keep in mind that, like with anything you'd purchase at a boutique-type store (like a yoga mat), you'll probably pay more for a ball at your local gym unless it comes with some kind of a health club discount.

While You're Out: Other Balls and Accessories to Consider

Personal trainers and physical therapists are using all kinds of new balls that come in different shapes and sizes. And even more intimidating, you can see all these different kinds of balls on ball racks at the gym. Even I get confused sometimes about knowing the differences between all these balls and how I'm supposed to use them!

Weighing the pros and cons of a heavy ball

Heavy balls, or weighted balls, are relatively new to the world of fitness. But just what are they? For starters, _heavy balls_ are smaller weighted medicine balls that range in weight from 1 pound to 12 pounds. They're versatile because they're hollow inside and are filled with water or sand, which offers a great alternative to hand weights and dumbbells.

You can use heavy balls to train for throwing and catching drills, squatting, lunging, and jumping. They provide a natural range of motion that helps improve your golf swing or enhance the swing of a bat that the clumsiness of dumbbells can't. Heavy balls are extremely effective for targeting the muscles in your upper body because their small, round shape allows you to use them through a full range of motion and improve your grip at the same time. Just gripping a heavy ball in your hand will incorporate the use of the small muscle groups in your hands and wrists. By developing these small muscles groups, heavy balls can help develop muscle coordination and improve reaction time through the use of throwing and passing drills.

Exchanging heavy balls for hand weights to do the exercises shown in Chapters 6 and 7 can be a fun and challenging way to incorporate these new accessories into your workout.

Heavy balls come in many different sizes, beginning with the smallest ones that are about the size of a tennis ball. The largest of the heavy balls is slightly bigger than a softball and are perfect for targeting the smaller muscle groups in your hands, arms, and upper body.

The following is a list of the heavy balls' attributes and what they can do for you (so you know the difference if you're going to use them or in case anyone asks you what the heck they are). Heavy balls

✔ Strength train and tone your upper body more than old-fashioned dumbbells because *grasping* them incorporates the smaller muscle groups located in your hands.

✔ Provide a more natural feel than dumbbells.

✔ Are water-filled or sand-filled, depending on the brand or manufacturer.

✔ Are color-coded to show weight differences. Most heavy balls come in green, red, yellow, blue and orange.

Green is the most widely used color because it's easy to grasp (about the size of a softball) and weighs only a little more than 1 pound.

✔ Are sized according to the size of your hands.

✔ Increase in size by one-inch increments in accordance to their weight; so the heavier they are, the larger they are.

Because of heavy balls' round shape, they're more fun to train with than hand weights. You can use them for power throws with a partner and squats, plus you certainly don't have to worry about getting rough or calloused hands like you do with hand weights. But you may have to worry about your heavy balls rolling away, so be sure you keep a good, tight grip!

For those who love gadgets and gizmos: Great new accessories

When you purchase your new ball, it probably will come with a catalogue of other products and fun accessories that you can use with it. These accessories can be anything from a faster, simpler air pump to a stability cushion that looks like a pancake, which you use to train your entire core.

What is a medicine ball?

A medicine ball, similar in shape and size to a basketball, is a unique tool that only training professional athletes once used. Considered to be very "old school," you probably saw the medicine ball featured in a lot of old movies where training boxers passed it back and forth. Nowadays, the medicine ball is quickly becoming a staple in gyms all over the world.

The medicine ball provides resistance through a full range of motion, like curling and pressing, and is superior to using weight machines that are bolted to the wall. Just like the exercise ball, the medicine ball helps strengthen the core muscles, which are where all our movements originate.

Medicine balls start at 1 pound and go up to 15 pounds. When combined with the exercise ball, the medicine ball becomes an amazing tool for a complete body workout. You can use it to strengthen your back, shoulders, arms, and legs as well as strengthen the entire core of your body (see Chapter 16 for exercises featuring the medicine ball).

Because the popularity of the ball is growing at such a rapid rate and is fast becoming the biggest trend in fitness, I list some of the most popular accessories that you can get and that I'm sure you'll be seeing at the gym if you haven't already!

- ✔ **Mini ball (20 cm):** This mini ball, sometimes called a Pilates ball, is most commonly used as a stress reliever. You place it between your upper back and the wall and roll up and down in a wall squat (as Chapter 9 shows) to relieve tension in your back.

- ✔ **Medicine balls (2 pounds up to 8 pounds):** Medicine balls are smaller balls that make ideal training tools by adding resistance without the use of cumbersome hand weights.

- ✔ **Stretching ball (75 cm):** This ball is made for stretching only and is larger than most exercise balls used for aerobics and strength training.

- ✔ **Ball net:** A ball net is made of a net-like material and has a handle, which you use to transport your ball anywhere you want to go — without it rolling out into the street!

- ✔ **Sit-n-Gym:** This accessory, also called a ball with legs, is great if you need extra support to balance on the ball. It has four small protrusions that act as "legs" for additional balancing on the ball. I recommend this one for seniors.

- ✔ **Ball base:** You use this base to store your ball in your home or at work, so you don't have to worry about your dog or cat hurting himself on the ball when you're not home. Or you may just want to know where your ball is at all times.

- ✔ **Carrying strap:** You can adjust this strap to any individual ball size for the added convenience of toting your ball with you wherever you go.

✔ **Ball stacker:** This accessory is a stacking system for multiple balls that keeps them secured in your home gym or office. Plus, a ball stacker keeps them looking nice and organized.

✔ **Plug puller:** This accessory looks like a corkscrew or a bottle opener, and you use it to pull the plug out of your ball for easier inflating (because that sucker can get stuck in there pretty good sometimes).

✔ **Physio Rolls:** This device is a peanut-shaped ball that gives you better control, and I highly recommend it for seniors because it provides more stability than the round exercise ball. This ball is sometimes called an "hourglass ball" because it's shaped just like an hourglass!

✔ **Air-pump adapter:** You add this device to an air compressor for faster ball inflation.

✔ **Balance disc:** This stability disc is a circular cushion you can use for standing, kneeling, or sitting to help you develop balance and coordination. The disc is made of a rubber-like material and looks like a pancake that's filled with air.

✔ **Firm ball:** This ball is 75 cm or larger and is firmer than a regular exercise ball. A firm ball provides additional durability and a more intense workout. It is a professional quality ball that makes workouts tougher by providing an extra firm base, which makes staying seated more difficult.

✔ **Ball chair:** You've probably heard of replacing your chair with the ball, but a ball chair is actually a chair that the ball fits right into. It looks like a regular chair with the seat cushion taken out, so the perfect ball size for you can fit right in. The ball chair provides more support for your back than just an exercise ball does by taking pressure off your spine while correcting your posture and improving your balance. Ball chairs also are available without backs, so they look like a circular frame (like something that would hold a globe). Ball chairs are also great for children, and they come in all sizes.

A ball by any other name . . .

Swiss ball, stability ball, exercise ball, gym ball, body ball, large ball, fitness ball, Resist-A-Ball, and now an aero ball? Whew! The ball goes by a lot of different names, doesn't it? And if you read this chapter, at least you know the difference between the exercise ball and a medicine ball or a heavy ball and a physio ball, right?

Whatever you choose to call the ball, its simple, round shape and fun, playful quality seems to be taking the world by storm. Not only does the ball provide you with a more comfortable environment for sitting and working out for whatever age group or demographic you're in, but it also offers elite athletes and back pain suffers tremendous benefits as well.

Oops! I just found another name I left out — a workout ball. Now, I wonder what that could be?

Chapter 3

Feeding and Caring for Your Ball

*F*illing your ball with air may seem simple until you spend 30 minutes with a hand pump and your ball still looks like a squash. And when you finally get your ball filled up to where you think it should be, it seems much too small! Because your new ball gradually loses air over time, you'll have to fill it up over and over again so it's just the right height. You can use anything that fills up a tire or an air mattress, but I suggest trying one of the products I list in this chapter to help you get a better and faster result.

This chapter covers the ABCs of how to fill your ball with air and how to care for it properly after you have it just right. I also cover some other safety concerns, like storing your ball somewhere out of the way and keeping it cool, in this chapter. So what are you waiting for? Let's get rolling.

What to Use to Inflate Your Ball

Every new ball comes with the manufacturer's instructions on how to fill it up according to the pump you're using. You can follow these instructions and then fine tune the procedure by reading this chapter or finding out if your neighbor owns an air compressor. But even if you're that fortunate, you don't want to fill your ball with too much air! I suggest reading on to find what you should know about rounding out your ball.

Hand pump

Most brands of balls are sold with small hand pumps about the size of your hand. It's true! These pumps are pretty small and make filling your ball with air a bit tedious. I've timed the filling process and, believe me, I didn't feel like working out when I was done. Whatever the case may be, these pumps do work, so don't forget where you put them when you're done filling up your ball.

If you purchase an exercise ball that doesn't include a hand pump, you can buy a pump that's especially for the ball. You can find such a pump at any sporting goods store for around $9. Among the choices that you can purchase are pumps that use *dual action*. Dual action means that the air pump works in both directions, giving you a quicker filling of your ball. You can use most dual-action pumps for all different types of balls, like medicine balls or basketballs, because they come with interchangeable nozzles or tips.

You can use a bicycle pump as long as it comes with an adapter that you can use to fill your ball with air.

Foot pump

Foot pumps range in size from 5 liters and up, and companies market them as being less stressful on your body. (I tend to agree and think that they're less stressful in general!) For anywhere from $9 to $45, you can purchase a foot pump through many of the Internet Web sites (see Chapter 2 for these sites).

Most manufacturers that sell their products online include foot pumps with their ball kits. Most manufacturers that sell their products in sporting goods or retail stores favor hand pumps. The reason is because kits sold in retail stores are marketed to the general public, whereas exercises balls sold online are marketed to personal trainers and physical therapists.

Don't expect your foot pump to look like one of those old bicycle tire pumps. This foot pump looks more like an air compressor with a small hose, and it works pretty well.

Air compressor

An air compressor or an air hose (like the one at your local gas station) is great for filling up your ball with air and is definitely faster than a foot pump or hand pump. If you do use the air hose at a gas station, be sure you don't fill up your ball too much with air and that you can fit it in your car for the ride home!

Online you can also purchase a time-saving adapter that you can attach to compressors or air hoses. The cost of an adapter is around $5. These products are great for filling your ball safely with air in seconds!

Filling Your Ball With Air: Tightness Versus Firmness

When you inflate your ball, you should inflate it to the diameter that the sizing instructions show. You want to fill the ball with air only until it feels like it has a slight give and it's not too taut or firm.

There's a big difference between filling your ball with air so it's tight like a drum and filling it with just enough air so that it's firm and stabilizing as it should be. Filling your ball with air is like striking the perfect balance when you purchase a new mattress to sleep on: You don't want it to be too hard, and you definitely don't want it to be too soft, either. Read on to find the best way to check your ball's air level so it feels just right for you.

When you first inflate your ball, it may seem too small. Give it at least 24 hours for the material to adapt to the expansion before you add more air to it.

Going for firmness

The general rule when you're filling the ball with air is that you want it to have a little give when you sit on it. However, you don't want it to be squishy or soggy. Your ball should feel firm and supportive but not tight like a drum.

If you look at yourself in the mirror when you're sitting on your ball, you should be able to see a slight indentation where the weight of your body is resting (as Figure 3-1 shows).

If your height to weight ratio is larger than it should be, you need to use a larger ball than the instructions prescribe for you because your extra weight will flatten out the ball when you sit on it. After you purchase a larger ball, under-inflate it until your feet are flat on the ground to adjust the level of firmness.

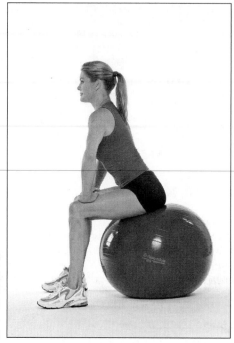

Figure 3-1:
Proper level
of firmness
for your ball.

Doing the bounce test

Besides sitting on the ball to test the air level, you can also give it the bounce test. After you've filled your ball with air, check the following list to see whether it meets all these requirements when you're bouncing on it:

✔ **Make sure that your feet are flat on the floor and that your weight is evenly distributed.** Both hips and sides of your body should be level with each other.

✔ **Make sure that your knees are level or slightly lower than your hips, creating a 90-degree angle.** Your thighs should be parallel to the ground or pointed down slightly.

✔ **Make sure that your hips, shoulders, and ears are all in a vertical line when you're sitting tall on the ball.** To test this function and to align yourself properly, try bouncing up and down lightly.

Adjusting your air levels

When you fill your ball with air, you'll find that your ball has some adjustability to it. In other words, you can adapt your ball to your own individual level of comfort.

If you find that your hips are much higher than your knees (as if you were sitting on a pillow that's on top of a chair), you can release some air until your knees and hips are level or slightly elevated. Also, if you use your ball regularly, expect your ball to lose pressure and to have to inflate it as necessary.

Keep in mind that if you do release air from your ball, it may cause your ball to lose air pressure, which actually makes the ball a more stable base because it'll be flatter and easier for you to sit on.

 When you become comfortable doing ball exercises, you want to make the ball a bit more taut to increase your level of training. The firmer the ball, the more difficult staying seated on it becomes because it requires more strength from your stabilizing muscles. You need to have stronger abdominal muscles just to keep the ball in place.

Keeping Your Ball Safe and Sound

Knowing how to keep your ball still and how to make it last for a long time are just a few of the things you want to consider when you bring your new ball home.

You should remember that exercise balls gradually lose air over time when just sitting around and that you should store them somewhere safe. In this section, I give you a few valuable tips that you can use to maintain your exercise ball and keep it from rolling off into the sunset.

Storing the ball

You can store your ball in a lot of ways and places now, thanks to the many new products that are on the market. (I guess someone finally discovered that balls like to roll away in any direction when you're not watching them.)

Whether you're in a group ball class or just working out on it around your house, an exercise ball can be a dangerous thing when combined with dogs, babies, hand weights, and other accessories. Plus, finding a storage area in your home that's safe and big enough for the ball can be challenging.

In the spirit of making your world a safer place, here are some of the following products available for keeping your ball out of the way:

- ✔ **A ball base:** A *ball base* is a circular black base that you can use to store your ball so you don't have to worry about your pets or other people hurting themselves when you're not around. You also can use it so you know where your ball is at all times. Group ball classes at gyms use these bases to rest the ball on while members use other pieces of equipment like resistance bands and hand weights. That way, class members don't have to worry about the ball getting away from them!

- ✔ **A ball stacker:** A *ball stacker* is a plastic stacking system that you can place one or more balls on to keep them secure and stabilized in your home or office. It fits neatly in any corner and keeps things looking nice and organized.

Keeping it away from extreme temps

Placing your ball next to a window isn't a good idea. Direct sunlight or extreme changes in temperature can erode the plastic or surface of your ball and cause it to expand. Also keep your ball away from other sources of heat, such as the furnace in your home, the clothes dryer, and any floor or ceiling vents, because the ball can expand from the sudden change in temperature. The same goes for cold temperature changes, which can cause the ball to expand and burst.

Be careful not to place your ball in any place that encounters extreme changes of temperature — either hot or cold. Doing so will help preserve your ball and keep its shape for a long time to come.

Wiping down the ball

Like with any piece of fitness equipment, you should wipe down your ball after a good workout for hygienic purposes, especially if you sweat a lot. If you've ever used an exercise mat in a group class at the gym, you know how badly they can smell after someone else has used them and forgotten to wipe them down.

The life of your ball

How long can you expect your ball to last? Well, that's all up to you, really. Here's a list of a few things that you can do to ensure that your ball will last for many, many years:

✔ Make sure that you purchase a quality ball (see Chapter 2) that holds 600 or more pounds.

✔ Make sure that your ball is anti-burst so if you puncture it, it will deflate slowly.

✔ Make sure that you wipe down your ball regularly so that lotions and other products don't erode the surface.

✔ Make sure that you don't overload the ball when you add weights to your workout so it surpasses the maximum weight requirement.

✔ Make sure that you check the air levels of your ball regularly to keep it properly inflated.

✔ Make sure that you store your ball properly away from any extreme changes in temperature.

If you do all these things to protect the surface of the ball and its shape, your ball can hang around forever.

Using regular soapy water instead of commercial cleaning product to keep the surface of your ball clean is best to ensure that the ball doesn't pick up any kind of chemical odor.

Checking air levels

Be sure to check your ball's level of air each time before you use it. Even if your ball just sits around not getting used, it loses air. So test your ball's air regularly by following the guidelines I provide earlier in this chapter in the section "Going for firmness."

Finding an open space

To play it safe when you use the ball for training, make sure you have some room to roll around — literally. If you're using it in a room in your house, find an open area or clear one that's at least 5 feet by 5 feet (or larger, depending on your height). Remove anything from the room that has sharp edges, like a coffee table or stereo, to keep from running (or rolling) into it when you exercise. And don't forget to check for any debris on the floor that could puncture or injure the ball.

Because you never know what direction the ball is going to roll in or what position you'll be using with any given exercise, be sure that you have enough room to lie flat on the floor with your arms extended over your head while you're holding the ball. If you have that much room, you should have enough space to move in any direction and stretch out properly on the floor.

Chapter 4

Gathering Your Gear and Getting Ready

As the old saying goes, Rome wasn't built in a day, so keep a positive attitude as you discover how to work out on the ball. Before you begin working out on the ball, though, you need to know how to *sit on it,* right?

Also, knowing what you need to work out on the ball ahead of time and knowing how much space it'll all take up is important because, after all, you're dealing with a large ball here. And that fact may be a little intimidating when you're just getting started. Read on to find out everything you should know before you start your workout so you can begin and end with a feeling of confidence. And by the time you reach the end if this book, I bet you'll be a pro . . . or just look like one!

Absolute Essentials

Okay, so you bought your ball. Is that all you need? Not really, if you want to check your posture, practice various exercises, and tone up with some hand weights. Using any or all these items can add up to big changes and help make your workout more successful and comfortable as you progress with the exercises.

Here's a little more information on a few accessories that are important to gather as you begin.

A mirror

Coming from a dance background, I'm used to using a mirror to check to see whether I'm lifting my chest properly, not bending my knees, and standing up straight. A mirror is a great tool for making sure that you have the desired neutral alignment of your spine on the ball (see the photos in this chapter) and throughout many of the exercises contained in this book.

So what kind of mirror works best? For starters, any mirror that's bolted to the wall! Because the ball rolls in all different directions, you don't want to use a free-standing mirror (like a wardrobe mirror). If you have the space in your garage or office, a wall mirror works great for checking your body alignment — and for staying put.

Exercise mat

Use an exercise mat in combination with the ball for these reasons:

- ✔ Because you have to kneel in many of the ball exercises, you need a mat to cushion your knees.

- ✔ Because you lie on the floor while performing many of the ball exercises, you need the mat underneath you to lie more comfortably on a hard surface.

- ✔ Because you can easily slip while you're working out on the ball, using a mat gives you better traction and makes keeping the ball underneath you easier.

- ✔ Whether you're lying down or face up on the ball, you need to keep a good grip on the floor with your feet, otherwise you may lose your balance and slip right off.

In addition, find a mat that's the right size for you. If you get a mat that's too small, when you lie on your back to perform your exercises, your head will hang off onto the floor. When you're buying a mat, follow these guidelines:

> ✔ If you're 5 feet tall, use a mat that's about 6 feet long to allow you room to lie flat and extend the ball over your head.
>
> ✔ If you're more than 5 feet 5 inches tall, get a 7-foot mat to allow for your extra height.

A towel

During a workout, I recommend having a towel to wipe down yourself and the ball because its surface can become quite slippery and unstable. Having a towel by your side at all times keeps the surface clean and dry.

You can also use a towel as a cushion for your knees and your back if you decide not to purchase an exercise mat. Make sure the towel you use is long enough for you to lie on when you're stretched out on the floor because many of the exercises in this book use this position. If you don't already have an oversized towel, you can find them at most department stores or you can use a beach towel.

When you're ready to work up a good sweat, you'll need to have a bottle of water handy so you can drink frequently to replace what you lose during the sweating process.

Adding Weights

Both men and women can benefit greatly from using weights to firm and tone up with just the right amount of weight. You can accomplish that feat by performing the ball exercises in this book with one of the following recommended types of weights.

Because the ball is an unstable base, lifting weights and trying to keep your balance is challenging. Never use weights that you can't lift without keeping a neutral alignment in your spine.

Keeping the ball steady and making sure that your feet remain on the floor at all times when lifting any amount of weight is important so you don't lose your balance and fall off the ball.

Hand weights

For women who want to increase their lean body mass and tone up and are comfortable and able to maintain their balance while working out on the ball, using weights that allow you to do 10 to 15 repetitions is just the right amount. Most women who are just starting out should use 3- to 5-pound weights.

For women who are already conditioned and in good shape, I recommend using 10- to 15-pound weights to get a more challenging workout.

Ankle weights

Adding ankle weights to floor exercises with the ball not only increases the intensity, but it also increases your level of fitness. Besides increasing the gravitational pull while exercising, the extra weight works your glutes, hamstrings, calves, and quadriceps for better toning and definition.

Most ankle weights start at 1½ pounds and go up to 15 pounds. The most popular and effective weight to use for starting out is between 2 and 10 pounds. Ankle weights that wrap around the ankle and can be adjusted to your individual size work best.

Dumbbells

For men and women who are interested in building muscle mass, heavier dumbbells that allow you to complete only six to eight repetitions comfortably are perfect. Most people can safely use 15 to 25 pounds with the ball without sacrificing proper form.

Heavy balls

Heavy balls are a good accessory to consider using to increase your resistance and to add some amount of weight to your workout (see Chapter 2). Heavy balls range in size from a tennis ball to a softball and start out weighing just less than a pound. They continue to increase in size in one-inch increments and are available in different colors to identify their weight and size. Heavy balls are easier to grip than hand weights because of their round shape and provide more overall toning for the smaller muscles located in the wrist and hands.

Why use resistance training?

Using different forms of resistance, such as hand weights and dumbbells, to reduce overall body fat has gotten a lot of attention lately. (I guess you cardio junkies need to take a break and read up on just a few of the reasons why a weight-training session burns more calories.)

Here are a few of the many benefits you get from resistance training:

✔ You burn 30 to 50 calories per day for each pound of muscle you put on.

✔ Building bigger muscles boosts your metabolic rate (the rate at which you burn calories) and reduces overall body fat.

✔ "Burn calories while you sleep?" Yes, it's true — lean body mass burns more calories than fat does. So if you have more muscle, you can burn more calories while you sleep.

✔ It improves your posture as a result of strengthening your back muscles, which help develop a long spine.

✔ It increases your strength and muscle mass, which reduces the risk of osteoporosis.

✔ It protects your joints and muscles from deterioration.

✔ It strengthens the connective tissue within your body.

To burn the most amount of calories in the shortest amount of time, you need to work the larger muscle groups in your body. Next time you're doing a workout, try a few of these compound exercises rather than exercises that target individual muscles:

✔ Squats

✔ Lat pulls

✔ Chest presses

These exercises are great examples of ways to burn the most calories in the shortest amount of time.

No weights

If you're pregnant or have back or neck injuries, only use the resistance that your individual body weight provides while on the ball.

If you're brand new to working out on the ball, I recommend not using weights because, although you may have strong muscles on the outside of your body, you probably need to strengthen your inside muscles (or core stabilizing muscles) first to develop control over all your movements.

Dressing for the Occasion

Although dressing for every kind of sport has become fashionable (rugby shirts and even tennis wear has become hip), here are some real safety considerations you need to keep in mind before getting on the ball. Because bare skin can stick to the sticky surface of the ball, covering up is best. You'll also sweat during your workout, which can cause you to slip off the ball when you're not wearing the proper attire. Here are a few tips to consider when dressing for your ball workout.

Wearing proper clothing

Because the ball is made of a rubbery material, wearing anything that's latex or slippery can make holding various positions difficult. Keeping your grip and being able to remain upright while seated on the ball is very important, so avoid wearing anything that's shiny or slick for your workout.

Wearing bulky clothes or untucked shirts can get caught on the ball or bunch up while you're working out, so stick with something form-fitting, like what you'd wear to a yoga class.

Accessories

Any kind of jewelry or zippers that can jab or bust your ball are obviously not a good idea. Earrings are especially dangerous when you turn your head to the side because they can poke the ball and bust it; if you have an anti-burst ball, they'll cause a slow leak.

Buckles and belts are hazardous for a couple of reasons. First, they can puncture the surface of the ball when you're lying face down on the ball. And second, they can also press into your body, which can force you to hold your breath (which you know is a no-no).

Do I need shoes?

Because you are in many different positions when exercising on the ball, you need to be able to grip the floor with your feet so you can steady yourself and keep your balance. If you have a pair of tennis shoes with good traction, wear those because they provide additional support for your ankles when you're bouncing or rolling in different directions. When you use hand weights and other accessories like medicine balls, you need your shoes to protect your toes in case you drop a weight on them! Ouch!

But when you're using an exercise mat and the ball for stretching, yoga, and Pilates, you may want to remove your shoes because the sticky surface of the mat provides enough protection from slipping off the ball.

In your bare feet, you're able to feel the support of the floor beneath you to better balance yourself and to get a better stretch. Plus, bare feet make maneuvering in and out of difficult positions easier than it is when you're wearing shoes.

Keeping your hair in check

I'm sure you've heard a horror story or two about someone who went on a roller coaster and got her hair got caught in the tracks. Yikes! Well, the same goes for the ball: Loose hair can be a safety hazard when you're draped over the ball or lying on your back because it can easily get caught underneath the ball and literally rolled over. Keeping your hair out of your face also gives you a clearer view of the direction you're headed in when you start rolling around and changing positions.

Picking the Right Place for Your Workout

Do you exercise in the living room on the carpet or in the office on the hardwood floor? Picking the right room and the right surface for working out makes all the difference in the world and can make or break your workout. Read on to find out more specifics about which space is best to roll around in.

How much space do I need?

Because you never know what direction the ball is going to roll in or what position you'll be using with any given exercise, be sure that you have enough room to lie flat on the floor with your arms extended over your head while holding the ball.

You'll also be standing with the ball above your head for some of the exercises, so you want to make sure that the space is tall enough to accommodate the ball when you're standing. This space allowance should be enough to permit you to move in any direction and stretch out properly on the floor.

If you're using a room in your house, find an open area or clear one that's at least 5 feet by 5 feet or 6 feet by 6 feet (if you're taller than 5 feet 8 inches). The general rule is two feet longer than your height and two feet wider than the width of your arms. (If you lie down and pretend you're making a snow angel, you can measure the space you need that way.)

Don't forget to remove anything with sharp edges from this space, like a coffee table or stereo, to keep from running or rolling into it when you exercise.

The best surface for your workout

I recommend using a safe, non-slip surface when working out on the ball so you don't have the additional danger of sliding around with the already-slippery surface of the ball.

The following is a list of a few types of surfaces you can choose and recommendations for each:

- ✔ **A laminate floor or kitchen flooring:** A big no-no! Steer clear of any type of sticky flooring that you clean with chemical cleaners because the ball can pick them up and transfer them to your body when you roll around. (I just picked a few dog hairs off my ball.) Yuck!

- ✔ **Carpeting:** You probably have carpeting in your living room and, after moving the coffee table, you probably have a pretty convenient, nice-size space to work with. If you're going to use the ball on carpet, you need to use shoes with really good traction so you stay put, because your feet will have a tendency to slip out from under you when you're seated on the ball.

I don't recommend using a mat underneath the ball when you're on carpet because, when you combine the slippery surface of the mat with the static surface of the carpet, it provides a hazardous combination. Think sled riding!

- ✔ **Hardwood floor:** At most gyms or fitness centers, you find a hardwood surface. If you use your ball at home on a hardwood floor, just make sure that it's free of splinters and dirt because they can puncture or accumulate on the ball. Also, definitely use a towel or exercise mat to cushion your knees from the hard surface of the floor.

Setting Aside Enough Time to Work Out

In every workout, make sure you include a warm-up that consists of 10 to 15 minutes of movement (see Chapter 5) to increase your core temperature and to prepare your body for the exercises that are about to come.

After you have finished working out, be sure to cool down properly (see Chapter 10) to stretch out any muscle tightness you may have and to reduce your risk of injury.

For your actual workout, strive for at least 30 minutes three times a week to start your new ball program. Because you use your deeper abdominal muscles (which you probably haven't used before) when you work out on the ball, your body will feel the difference right away and be a bit sore throughout your core (from your ribs to your hips). Resting for 48 hours between workouts gives your body a chance to replenish and recharge. If you still feel some soreness after you rest for 48 hours in between your workouts, I recommend working a different part of your body or a different muscle group entirely to prevent any damage to the area. Make sure you drink a lot of water to aid in tissue repair, and try gentle stretching on the ball until you feel ready to start again.

As you become more proficient on the ball, you can increase your workouts to 60 minutes three to four days a week. The saying "you get out of it what you put into it" applies here, like anything in life that's worthwhile.

Adding short ten-minute cardio workouts, like jumping rope, on the days that you're not using the ball provides you with faster results and gives your metabolism a boost to burn extra calories.

Getting to Know Your Ball

When you first get your ball, start by sitting on it and familiarizing yourself with the sensation of contracting your abdominal muscles to keep your balance. Doing so may seem unnatural to you at first — which is perfectly normal, because when was the last time you sat on a ball and not a chair? The first thing you need to know is how to sit on the ball so your spine is in neutral alignment with the rest of your body and your feet are flat on the floor. Before you begin working out on the ball, take a look at the following photos to see how and where you need to sit on the ball.

Trying seated positions

Your pelvis can move in three distinct ways when you're sitting on the ball, and those ways are as follows: neutral, anterior, and posterior. But only one of those ways is the *correct* way to sit on the ball when you're trying to improve your posture, enhance your balance, and draw on your stabilizing muscles for support.

Throughout this book, I mention neutral spine to remind you just how important holding this position is when you're sitting on the ball. (For more on neutral spine, see Chapter 12 on Pilates.)

Neutral position

When you're seated on the ball, the correct position you want to be in is called the *neutral position*. To try the neutral position, follow these steps and check out the photo:

1. **Sit tall on the ball with your feet shoulder-width apart.** Make sure that your shoulders and ears are in line with each other.

2. **Lift your chest and draw your shoulder blades back and down, pinching them slightly together.**

3. **Place your hands on your knees or on either side of the ball for support.** Your legs should be even or parallel to the floor.

4. **Hold your back straight and long so that your pelvis is neither rolling forward nor backward; your pelvis should point straight down to the ground (as Figure 4-1 shows).**

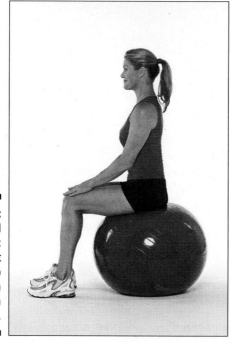

Figure 4-1: Neutral position: the correct position to use when seated on the ball.

Make sure you maintain the natural curve in your back by inhaling deeply and pulling your shoulder blades back as you lift your chest up toward the ceiling.

Here are a few do's and don'ts when in the neutral position:

✔ *Do* keep both feet on the floor at all times.

✔ *Do* tighten your abdominal muscles (or set your abdominals) for support.

✔ *Don't* hold your breath; breathe deeply and comfortably for better control.

✔ *Don't* forget to keep your feet shoulder-width apart. Bringing your feet closer together shortens your base of support and makes exercising more difficult.

If you feel unsteady or if you can't control the ball, place it against a wall or a heavy couch for support.

Anterior tilt

The *anterior tilt* is when you arch your back (which for most people is a comfortable position). Arching your back places unneeded pressure on your hip joints and strains your lower back.

In order to see how the anterior tilt position feels and to compare it to the neutral position, follow these steps:

1. **Sit tall on the ball with your feet shoulder-width apart.**

   Make sure that your shoulders and ears are in line with each other.

2. **Lift your chest and draw your shoulder blades back and down, pinching them together slightly.**

3. **Place your hands on your knees or on either side of the ball for support.**

   Keep your legs even with or parallel to the floor.

4. **Tilt your pelvis back slightly until you feel the arch in your spine (see Figure 4-2).**

Here are some do's and don'ts when trying the anterior position:

✔ *Do* maintain a long spine and sit tall on the ball.

✔ *Don't* forget to keep your hands on your knees or touching the ball on both sides of your body.

✔ *Don't* hold this position too long because it may make your back sore.

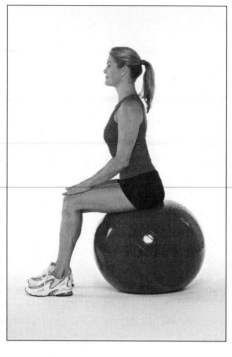

Figure 4-2:
Anterior tilt:
an incorrect
position to
use when
seated on
the ball.

Posterior tilt

You're in the *posterior tilt* when you roll your pelvis forward and your rib cage comes down toward your knees. In this position, you don't use any of your back muscles to lengthen and straighten your spine and allow your chest to sink toward the floor.

In order to see how the posterior tilt position feels and to compare it to the neutral position, follow these steps and check out the photo:

1. **Sit tall on the ball with your feet shoulder-width apart.**

   Make sure that your shoulders and ears are in line with each other.

2. **Lift your chest and draw your shoulder blades back and down, pinching them together slightly.**

3. **Place your hands on your knees or on either side of the ball for support.**

   Keep your legs even with or parallel to the floor.

4. **Roll your pelvis slightly forward until you feel your chest sink and your shoulders move inward toward your body (as Figure 4-3 shows).**

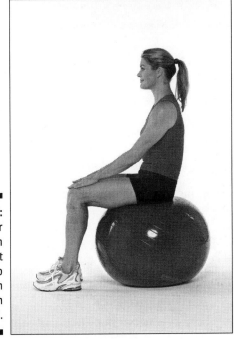

Figure 4-3:
Posterior
tilt: an
incorrect
position to
use when
seated on
the ball.

A few do's and don'ts when trying this position:

- ✔ *Do* roll slowly forward to keep from sliding sideways off the ball.

- ✔ *Don't* forget to keep both feet flat on the floor when you roll your pelvis forward.

- ✔ *Don't* add any arm movements when you're in this position because they may cause you to lose your balance.

Trying a seated bounce position

Besides tilting your pelvis forward and back a few times to get acquainted with sitting on the ball, you can try bouncing lightly up and down to see whether or not you've positioned yourself correctly and whether or not your weight remains centered.

To do this exercise, follow these steps:

1. **Sit tall on the ball with both feet flat on the floor, making sure that you evenly distributed your weight.**

Try to keep your hips and both sides of your body level with each other.

2. **Line up your hips, shoulders, and ears so that they're all in a vertical line.**

3. **Place your hands on either side of you and rest them lightly on the ball.**

4. **Bounce up and down slightly, keeping your feet flat on the floor at all times.**

5. **Stop bouncing periodically to see where your weight falls when the ball isn't in motion. Your weight should be centered straight up and down, and your back and spine should be long and tall.**

You should feel your pelvis pointing straight toward the floor as you bounce softly up and down on the ball.

Trying a supine position

When you lie with your back on the ball and your chest faces the ceiling, you're in the *supine position* (sometimes called *lying supine*). In this position, you support your weight with only your upper body because your hips and lower back aren't on the ball.

The *bridge exercise* is a really good example of lying in the supine position on the ball. In the bridge exercise, your hips press up toward the ceiling and your shoulders and upper back remain on the ball.

To do this exercise, follow these steps:

As you lift your hips up, keep your back from sagging or arching.

1. **Rest your head and shoulders on the ball with your knees bent at a 90-degree angle.**

   Make sure that you keep your knees stacked over your ankles.

2. **Press your hips toward the ceiling as high as possible (see Figure 4-4).**

3. **Slowly lower your hips back to the starting position.**

To strengthen and increase the load on your hips and lower back, try adding an extra press up with your butt.

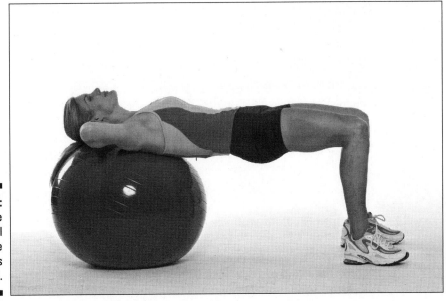

Figure 4-4:
Lying supine
on the ball
(otherwise
known as
the bridge).

A few do's and don'ts for this exercise:

- *Do* rest the back of your head on the ball during this exercise.

- *Don't* let your thighs and butt sink toward the ground; keep everything tight and pressed up during this exercise.

Perfect Fit: Positioning on the Ball

Many different parts of your body work to keep you steady on the ball. For starters, you have to use your back to maintain your posture so you stay seated on the ball. Then you need proper foot placement; without it, you'd fall on your tushy. Which brings us to the safety concerns that you need to be aware of when working out on the ball.

All the previous elements are important because they add up to your success and safety and make the ball a perfect fit for you. Read on to find out what you need to know to pull them all together.

Posture

In the world of fitness and dance, everyone learned that maintaining a "straight" back that had no arch in it at all was best. I remember having to press my back down to the floor to make sure it didn't lift up at all during dance class. Nowadays, doctors know that maintaining the slight natural arch in your back is best; in other words, you want a "long, tall spine."

The technical term for the natural curve in your spine is called the *lumbar lordosis*. Keeping this curve is good not only for exercising but also to maintain throughout the day.

If you have difficulty seeing and feeling a long spine, try this exercise:

1. **Lie on the floor with your back pressed down. If your back is flat, you shouldn't be able to put your hand between the floor and your back.**

2. **Now relax and lie comfortably for a moment as you place your hand on the small of your back (lower back) and feel the slight lift or arch that exists.**

3. **Exhale as you slowly bring your knees to your chest, still focusing on the placement of your back on the floor.**

4. **Hold your knees into your chest for a few moments, and then release your legs back to the floor.**

When you lie comfortably on your back in a resting position, you should feel the natural curve in your spine.

Feet placement

One of the most important elements of keeping steady and staying stable during your workout is the placement of your feet. Whenever you're seated on the ball, you need to keep both feet planted on the ground, unless you're doing an exercise that calls for you to carefully lift one leg off the floor. You should always have your feet directly under your knees, and you should always stack your knees directly over your ankles, creating a 90-degree angle.

Because the exercises require you to walk your feet forward (out in front of you) for many of the abdominal exercises, starting in a secure seated position is always important before beginning any movement.

Keeping your safety in mind

For the safest and most effective workout on the ball, follow these simple and easy tips:

- ✔ **Use a smooth and steady motion for each exercise.** When you're doing any form of resistance training, maintaining control is important. Whether you're lifting weights or doing resistance work on the ball, controlling the movement — and not letting the movement control you — is the key. If you start to lose your form, you're doing your body a disservice and you may injure yourself.

- ✔ **Breathe freely while exercising.** Never hold your breath while working out on the ball. Breathing freely helps you gain better control of the ball.

- ✔ **Remember to stay within your own limits.** Never try an exercise that may risk you hurting yourself on the ball.

- ✔ **Always check your ball's air level and make sure that your ball is in good working order before you begin your workout.** Never use a ball that's too low in air or that's over-inflated because it can make your workout much more difficult and cause you injury.

- ✔ **If you feel any kind of pain — especially in your joints — never continue the exercise.** Remember that a sharp pain is different from the slight pain or fatigue that you feel in your muscles when you're "going for the burn." Some exercises in this book may just not feel right for your particular body, so move on to find the ones that do.

- ✔ **Perform the exercises in this book only in the ways in which they're demonstrated.** Adding your own little twist to proven and effective exercises can cause injury or cause you to fall right off the ball and onto your tailbone. Ouch!

- ✔ **Stay within your training range.** When you begin working out after taking a long time off, going a little nutty and doing too much is easy to do. When you're just beginning, staying within your own level of comfort and not lifting too heavy a load keeps you from getting an injury and hindering your progress. If you're consistent with your exercise program, you'll see results in a few short weeks.

- ✔ **If you feel dizzy or short of breath, stop the exercise.** Because ball exercises use several positions where your head is lower than your heart (the drape), you can become dizzy from all the blood running downward. If you experience dizziness or shortness of breath, stop immediately and breathe deeply while you rest.

- ✔ **Exercise in an open space.** Never exercise in a confined or limited space. Remember to remove anything with sharp edges from your workout area to keep yourself from running or rolling into it when you exercise.

> ✔ **Always consult your doctor to make sure that you're in good physical shape before you begin a new exercise program.** In addition, if you have a history of back or neck problems or are pregnant, discuss these issues with your healthcare provider to find out if he or she feels that the ball is a good choice for you.

In addition, remember to always warm up properly to get your body ready for exercising and to avoid injury. And when you're finished working out, cool down to avoid soreness.

If You're the Classy Type

If you're anything like me, you'll do anything to find a good class. Whether it's kickboxing, spinning, or yoga, I find being in a group class very motivating. Okay, so maybe I just get bored when I'm on the elliptical trainer or the treadmill and am forced to watch Jerry Springer re-runs. Or maybe I just don't have the discipline to go it alone. But whatever the case may be, group ball classes are all the rage right now, so I suggest trying one as soon as you can!

Here are a few answers to some of the most frequently asked questions about what you should know when you do find a group ball class:

> ✔ **Where can I take a class?** Your local YMCA or YWCA is a good place to start looking for a group ball class. Local gyms and recreational centers also offer classes on a regularly scheduled basis, depending on the area you live in. You can call your local chamber of commerce to get a list of the fitness facilities in your area that offer exercise ball classes or search the Internet for a particular location.

> ✔ **How much does a ball class cost?** Ball classes range in price from $7 to $12 a class, depending on the facility that's offering them. If you're a member of a gym that offers ball classes, the cost is most likely included in your monthly payment.

> ✔ **Do I bring my own ball?** No. Group ball classes include balls of various heights for participants to use in the program. Getting to class early is important so you ensure that the right size ball is still available for you to use.

> ✔ **How long does the class take?** Ball classes frequently last 60 minutes. Classes begin with a warm-up and end with a cool down, so your actual workout time on the ball is 40 minutes. Many classes combine the exercise ball with other pieces of equipment, like medicine balls and resistance bands.

Some classes incorporate the ball along with other forms of training; these classes are called *circuit classes*. These classes add equipment like body bars, dumbbells, and cardio equipment like jump ropes to strengthen your body and increase endurance. Circuit classes are also known as boot camp classes because that's just what they are — tough, like a boot camp!

✔ **What kind of teacher should I look for?** Look for a teacher who can teach at all different levels, ranging from beginners to experienced athletes. Because the ball is unstable equipment, the teacher should be particularly conscientious of the level of his or her class to make sure that everyone in the class is using proper form at all times.

Health club providers usually require their instructors to have certifications, including ones from the International Sports Sciences Association, America Council on Exercise, Aerobics and Fitness Association of America, among others. Resist-A-Ball certifies instructors for core training that consists of different levels and other applications of the ball that they can use with Pilates, yoga, and pregnancy workouts.

✔ **What size class can I expect?** Ball classes vary in size each week according to attendance. Twenty-five is the maximum number of exercise balls available for most classes. "Series of classes" or "guaranteed classes" are offered at some fitness centers, whereas most gyms offer classes that are open to all members, which can greatly impact the size of the class.

✔ **How many times per week should I take a class?** To get the best results, taking a ball class two or three times per week is best. You should combine your ball classes with some form of cardio workout, which you can do on your days off from your group class. Walking, jumping rope, spinning, using the treadmill and an elliptical trainer are all perfect complements to using the ball.

Finally, here are some friendly group exercise reminders to make the transition into a ball class go a little smoother:

✔ Because some classes require participants to sign up ahead of time, always arrive early to make sure that you have a spot.

✔ Always arrive a few minutes early to class to give yourself time to select the right size ball for you.

✔ Never enter a class after the warm-up has begun because your body won't be well prepared for that particular workout.

Part II
Workouts to Have a Ball With

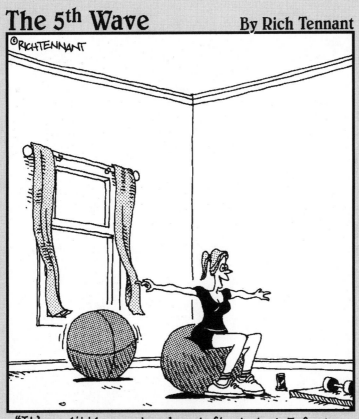

The 5th Wave   By Rich Tennant

"It's a little unsteady at first, but I feel completely stable now. How about you, Russell? Russell?"

In this part . . .

The exercises in Part II work your entire body. Starting with a fast-paced warm-up, this part moves into workouts for the shoulders and upper back (Chapter 6); arms (Chapter 7); chest, abdominals, and lower back (Chapter 8); and butt, hips, and legs (Chapter 9). At the end of these workouts, you cool down and stretch (Chapter 10), which leaves you feeling confident that you got a full-body workout.

And, if you're not too tired after all that work, this part takes you through a total body workout (Chapter 11) that will keep you tight and toned for good. I promise!

Chapter 5

Warming Up Your Body

. . . .

In This Chapter

▶ Knowing how and why to properly warm up your body

▶ Figuring out how to set your abs before warming up and working out

▶ Warming up on and off the ball

. . . .

*I*n this chapter, I give you a three-part warm-up routine that you can use to prepare for any of the workouts in this book. In addition, you can use this routine to warm up before any other types of exercise, too, such as walking, running, weight training, and so on.

In the first part of the warm-up, you start out on the ball with a few bounces in different proposed sequences. The next part takes you off the ball and gets you moving so you warm up your muscles and increase your heart rate. The final part of the warm-up puts you back on the ball to stretch and limber you up for whatever workout is in front of you. This routine should take about 15 to 20 minutes and, by the time you finish, your heart rate should be above 108 beats per minute.

To check your pulse rate, stop exercising and place your middle and index fingers around your wrist or on the side of your neck just below your jaw line. Look at the clock or your watch and count your pulse for 10 seconds; multiply that number by 6 to get the number of beats per minute. (And just for the sake of comparison, the average resting heart rate for an adult is 60 to 100 beats per minute.)

Use slow and controlled movements with each exercise and keep the number of your repetitions low (10 repetitions instead of 15) to warm up gradually instead of increasing your heart rate too fast. As always, if you're new to working out, consult your physician before you begin.

Do I Really Need to Warm Up?

To answer this question simply, *yes*. You really do need to warm up. A warm-up may consist of many different activities and exercises, but you need to do something that literally warms up your body. Launching into an exercise class as you run into the gym or going for a run right after lying on the couch can throw your body into shock and have serious consequences. If you don't warm up properly you can experience dizziness, fainting, fatigue, and nausea.

Slowly warming up your body encourages good circulation and gears you up for all the activity that you're about to do. In addition, being in the right frame of mind prepares you for a better workout and helps you concentrate and relax during the, shall we say, opening act?

First Things First: Setting Your Abs

Working out on the ball is different from sitting in a chair because the surface is round and uneven. At first, this difference may not seem like too big of a deal to you but, in reality, it is! The round surface of the ball enables you to engage your abdominal muscles and use your stabilizing muscles to keep from falling off. To have control over your balance and coordination and to master the exercises in this book, you need to practice, so expect to spend a bit of time doing so!

Before you begin any workout chapter in this book, you need to know how to do the following exercise to stay seated on the ball. By tightening your abdominal muscles and keeping your spine long and straight (*setting your abs*), you develop strength throughout the core muscles in your body and develop an awareness of where your movements originate.

Follow these steps to set your abs each time you get on the ball:

1. **Sit tall on the ball with your feet hip-distance apart and firmly planted on the ground.**

2. **Take a deep breath and visualize a belt tightening around your waist.**

3. **Let your rib cage lift and fill with air.**

4. **Place one hand below your belly button to feel the tightening and lifting.**

5. **Place your other hand on the small of your back to feel the natural curve of your spine as you're sitting tall on the ball.**

6. **As you exhale, keep your hand below your belly button to make sure your abs remain tight.**

When you set your abs properly, your body should feel as though it were ready for anything — like someone were going to punch you in the stomach and you're bracing yourself for the punch.

After a while, setting your abs becomes second nature to you. You'll immediately see the difference in your posture and in how you move throughout your day.

Holding your breath during any form of exercise, though it's a natural tendency for some people when they're trying a new form of exercise, is never a good idea. Make sure you don't hold your breath when you're working out on the ball because, as soon as you let it out, you may lose your balance. Breathing freely helps you keep your balance better and supplies oxygen to your muscles.

Warming Up on the Ball

Bouncing on the ball, marching, and stepping sequences are just a few of the many different exercises you can do on the ball to raise your core temperature and get your circulation going.

The following warm-up exercises will help you become familiar with bouncing up and down on the ball and help you achieve balance as you lift your legs and knees. Have fun!

Bouncing

I love those balls with the handles where you can leapfrog around the room or roll down a hill. Although the exercise ball doesn't have handles, it serves as a small trampoline that enables you to do small bounces up and down by lifting your body weight off it and returning back down to its round surface. The only difference between the exercise ball and one with the handles is that on the exercise ball, you have to use your center of gravity and your hands to guide you as you do small bounces.

The bouncing motion for this exercise will come naturally once you lift your weight off the ball and return back down to be greeted by the ball's round surface. If you were trying this exercise on a weight bench, it would hurt because you'd be greeted by a hard surface. Ouch!

Try placing the ball against a wall or heavy object, such as a couch, to keep the ball from moving when you jump up and come back down.

To do this exercise, follow these steps:

1. **Sit tall on the ball, keeping your hands at the sides of your body.**

2. **Lift up with your legs using a slight jumping motion as you straighten your knees (as Figure 5-1a shows).**

   Your hands will be off the ball and at your sides.

3. **Return to starting position, placing your hands back onto the ball for support (see Figure 5-1b).**

Complete a series of 10 to 15 bounces before beginning the next set of bounces. Do five sets of bounces in all.

A couple of do's for this exercise:

✔ *Do* use your leg and butt muscles to lift you off the ball rather than your hands.

✔ *Do* keep your movements small. You're bouncing, not jumping.

Figure 5-1:
Bounce
yourself into
a frenzy!
(Well, you
probably
don't need
to go *that*
far.)

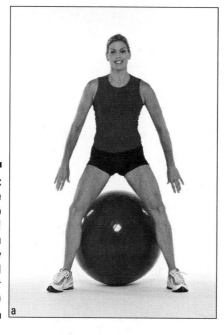
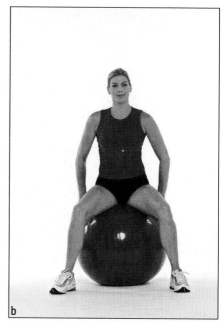

a
b

Heel touches

The object of this exercise is to keep the ball still as you reach out with your leg and alternate touching your heels to the floor. Believe me, this exercise isn't as easy as it looks!

To do this exercise, follow these steps:

1. **Sit tall on the ball with your feet shoulder-width apart and your hands at your sides.**

   Your hands will lightly touch the ball for support.

2. **Reach out with your right heel as you extend your right leg in front of you (see Figure 5-2).**

3. **Return your right heel to the starting position before you extend your left leg and heel to the opposite side.**

Alternate heel touches for two sets of 10 to 15 repetitions.

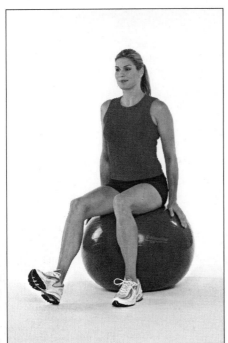

Figure 5-2:
Heel
touches.

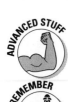

If you feel comfortable and balanced on the ball, try speeding up the movement.

A couple of do's and don'ts for this exercise:

- ✔ *Do* keep your back straight as you reach out and place your heel on the ground in front of you.
- ✔ *Don't* let both your feet leave the ground at the same time. Always keep one foot down on the floor.

Marching

Marching is a fun exercise when you do it on the ball. The key to this exercise is to raise your knees as high as possible without losing your balance and falling backward off the ball.

To make moving to the beat as you march more fun, turn on some music with a fast-paced tempo or drum rhythm.

To do this exercise, follow these steps:

1. **Sit tall on the ball with your feet shoulder-width apart and your hands at your sides.**
2. **As you tighten your stomach muscles for support, lift your right leg as high as possible (as Figure 5-3 shows).**
3. **Alternate lifting both legs in a marching fashion.**

Continue marching for a few minutes until you've warmed up your hips and are ready to go.

A few do's and don'ts for this exercise:

- ✔ *Do* keep your knees facing straight out in front of you, not out to the side.
- ✔ *Do* keep your hands on either side of you on the ball for support.
- ✔ *Don't* let the ball move. Keep it as still as possible.

Side stepping

By reaching with alternate legs while on the ball, the side step simultaneously opens up your pelvis and works your legs.

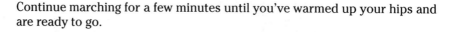

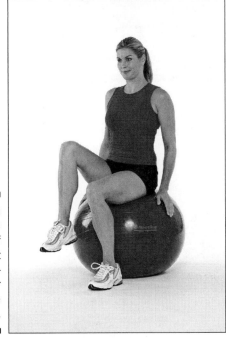

Figure 5-3:
March to
the beat of
a different
drummer —
or your
favorite
song.

To prevent falling off the ball, sit up straight and maintain perfect posture for this exercise.

To do this exercise, follow these steps:

1. **Sit tall on the ball and place your hands to your sides.**

2. **Extend your right leg out and to the side, straightening your right knee (as Figure 5-4a shows).**

3. **Slowly bring in your right leg and extend your left leg out to the opposite side (see Figure 5-4b).**

Complete 15 repetitions. You should do five sets in all.

A few do's and don'ts for this exercise:

✔ *Do* keep your hands behind your body and to your sides for support.

✔ *Do* straighten your leg as far as possible as you extend it to the opposite side.

✔ *Don't* lean forward on the ball when you step out with your alternating leg. Keep your back straight and lifted.

Flexibility: A man's problem?

The hamstrings, hips, and back are the tightest areas in the body, particularly for men. The reason is because men's bodies are primarily made up of muscle mass, whereas women's bodies are primarily made up of fat. Women have a greater fat composition, which is what ultimately separates the girls from the boys — a little bit of body fat in all the right places (that's what gives us women that great curve appeal). And let's face it, women are much more flexible as a result of that extra padding, but most guys I know can't even touch their toes!

Whether you're a man or a woman, properly warming up the body to increase your core temperature and increase your flexibility is essential. Before you begin a workout, enhance your flexibility and get your circulation going by starting out with five to ten minutes on the treadmill at a moderate speed or using the ball to perform ball bounces as shown in this chapter. Doing so better prepares your body for exercise and gets your heart rate up slowly.

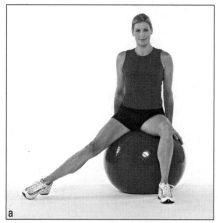 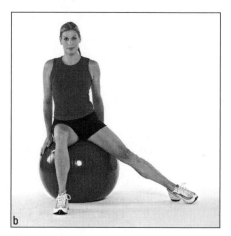

Figure 5-4:
Side
stepping.

a   b

Warming Up off the Ball

For the next part of the warm-up routine, you get to take a little break from sitting on the ball. You'll be on the ball for most of your workout, so you'll probably appreciate this part.

Now's the time to get on your feet and get your heart pumping!

Side circles

In this exercise, you use a big sweeping motion to get your heart rate up quickly. Remember to warm up slowly, though, and to use a controlled motion when swinging the ball from side to side. Believe me, doing side circles is harder than it looks!

The key to this exercise is to *plie,* or bend your knee out slightly to the sides, making room for the ball to move freely.

To do this exercise, follow these steps:

1. **Lift the ball above your head to start; then sweep the ball down toward the floor to one side of your body (as Figure 5-5a shows).**

   Keep your body loose so you can move the ball around easier while your back is straight for support.

2. **Sweep the ball down toward the floor to the opposite side of your body (see Figure 5-5b).**

Complete five repetitions.

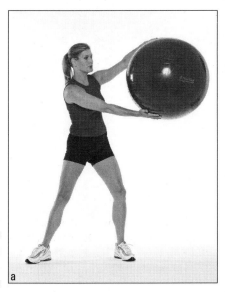
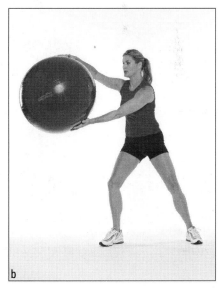

Figure 5-5:
Side circles.

Some do's and don'ts for this exercise:

✔ *Do* keep a firm grip on the ball to keep it from flying out of your grasp.

✔ *Do* inhale and exhale in unison with the swinging motion of your arms to help your body warm up more efficiently.

✔ *Don't* forget to bend your knees slightly and to keep your back straight as you move the ball from side to side.

Far-reaching ball squats

Far-reaching ball squats are great because they combine a squatting position with the extra weight of your upper body and the ball.

Make sure you keep your feet wider than shoulder-width apart so the ball can fit between your legs.

To do this exercise, follow these steps:

1. **Stand with your feet wider than shoulder-width apart and hold the ball as far above your head as you can (as Figure 5-6a shows).**

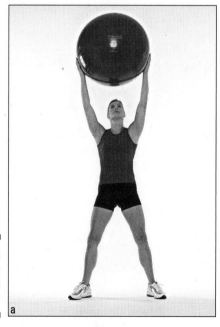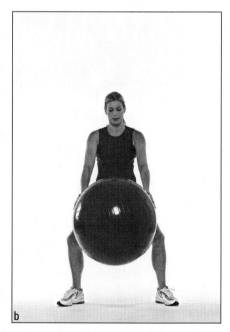

Figure 5-6:
Far-reaching ball squats.

a   b

2. **Keep your back straight as you lower the ball toward the floor using a squatting motion (see Figure 5-6b).**

3. **Use your heels to press your body back up into a standing position as you raise the ball above your head.**

Complete five to ten repetitions.

A few do's and don'ts for this exercise:

✔ *Do* keep your back straight as you squat down with the ball.

✔ *Do* gaze in the direction of the ball.

✔ *Don't* let the ball touch the floor when you lower it down.

Side lunges

This exercise combines a lunging motion with a slight roll of the ball. It's one of many cardio combinations that you can do with the ball to really stretch out your hamstrings, quads, and butt while increasing your heart rate.

To do this exercise, follow these steps:

1. **Bend one knee to the side in a lunge position and place the ball in front of your body within arm's reach.**

   Your back arm will be resting on your thigh for support.

2. **Lunge from side to side, rolling the ball to the opposite side of your body each time (as Figure 5-7 shows).**

Complete ten repetitions on each side.

For a more intense workout, try adding a few far-reaching ball squats in between the side lunges.

A few do's and don'ts for this exercise:

✔ *Do* keep the ball in front of you at arm's length so you can control it as you roll it from side to side.

✔ *Do* reach across your body using your opposite arm and leg.

✔ *Don't* let your knee move beyond your toe when you lunge from side to side.

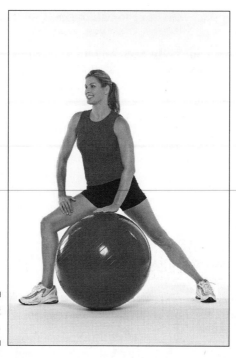

Figure 5-7:
Side lunges.

The Perfect Ending: Getting Back on the Ball

Okay, back on the ball! This next series of exercises uses a seated position on the ball and ends with a good back stretch. After this final part of the warm-up, you're ready for any workout.

Side reaches

Side reaches stretch the side muscles that run along your rib cage and help loosen up your entire body for a workout.

To do this exercise, follow these steps:

1. Sit tall and slightly forward on the ball.

2. **Roll the ball to the right, keeping your right leg perpendicular to the floor and extending your left leg behind you. Reach over your head with your left arm (see Figure 5-8).**

   Keep your right hand on your thigh to support your weight on the ball.

3. **Straighten back up, lifting from your obliques (your side muscles).**

4. **Repeat on the opposite side.**

Complete five reaches for each side.

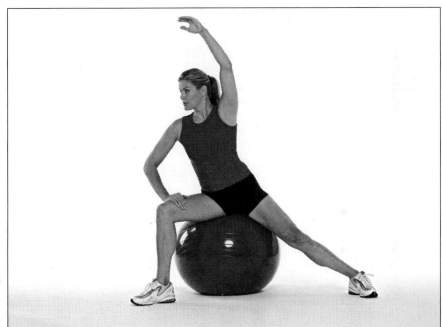

Figure 5-8:
Side reach.

A few do's and don'ts for this exercise:

- ✔ *Do* sit slightly forward on the ball, which makes getting a complete stretch easier.
- ✔ *Don't* reach too far to the side; you may lose your balance.
- ✔ *Don't* forget to exhale as you reach to the side.

Hip circles

Hip circles help loosen up the pelvis by releasing any built-up tension in the hip joint. To do this exercise, follow these steps:

1. **Sit tall on the ball with your feet shoulder-width apart (as Figure 5-9a shows).**

2. **With your arms at your sides, slowly circle your hips to the right, pressing the ball into the ground (see Figure 5-9b).**

3. **Repeat two or three circles to the right, and then repeat the exercise on the left side.**

Complete five repetitions on each side.

Some do's and don'ts for this exercise:

✔ *Do* circle your hips slowly to loosen up your entire hip and pelvic area.

✔ *Don't* let your feet leave the ground at any time during this exercise.

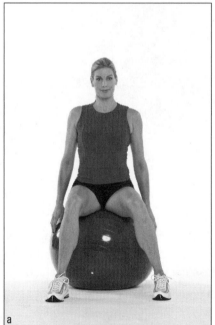 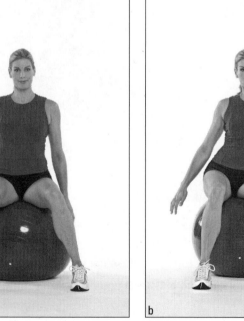

Figure 5-9:
Hip circles.

a

b

Chest and back stretch

This stretch helps release the back and the chest muscles at the same time. To do this exercise, follow these easy steps:

1. **Sit tall on the ball with your feet hip-width apart.**

2. **Bring your arms in front of you at chest level and clasp your hands together as you gently round your back (as Figure 5-10a shows).**

   Make sure that your eyes look down at the floor so your neck stays relaxed and in line with your spine.

3. **Slowly roll the ball forward to get an additional stretch in your lower back.**

4. **To reverse this stretch, open your arms and take them behind you as you roll the ball back slightly (see Figure 5-10b).**

5. **Stretch your chest by arching your spine gently.**

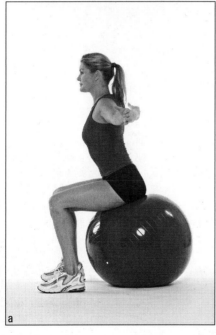 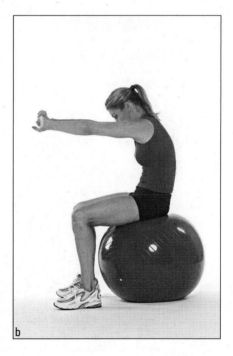

Figure 5-10:
Chest and back stretch.

A few do's and don'ts to keep in mind:

- ✔ *Do* breathe during this exercise to increase the stretch.
- ✔ *Do* keep your feet flat on the floor throughout the exercise.
- ✔ *Don't* rush this stretch. Take your time to relax and rejuvenate.

Back roll-up

I like to end my warm-up and workouts by rolling up my body one vertebrae at a time with this back roll exercise. The back roll-up helps loosen your upper back muscles, so take your time and roll up slowly.

Are you in your training zone? How to use a heart rate monitor

According to the U.S. Department of Health and Human Services, less than ten percent of the population exercises three or more times a week at a level vigorous enough to improve cardiovascular fitness and burn more calories than they take in. Because your heart rate is the most accurate measurement of how hard you're working while exercising and at rest, I suggest using a heart rate monitor. You can use this device as a personal coach to monitor your workouts.

Using a heart rate monitor is also a good way to check your pulse rate to make sure that you're properly warmed up. To find out whether your body's warmed up, take your age and subtract it from 220; then multiply the result by 0.60 (or 60 percent).

So if you're 40 years old, the math would look like the following:

$$220 - 40 = 180$$

$$180 \times 0.60 = 108 \text{ beats per minute}$$

To find your perfect training range, subtract your age from 220 and then multiply that number by 0.80 (or 80 percent). So, in this case:

$$220 - 40 = 180$$

$$180 \times 0.80 = 144$$

This number is your maximum heart rate for training within your zone (which is between 60 and 80 percent of your target heart rate) to improve your cardiovascular health and strengthen your heart.

In addition, most heart rate monitors have high and low signals or alarms that sound if you're out of your training range. They're as easy to read as a wristwatch and, when you purchase one, the salesperson can explain how to find your own personal training zone with it.

To do this exercise, follow these steps:

1. **Sit on the ball with your hands on your thighs and look straight ahead (as Figure 5-11a shows).**

2. **Keeping your back straight, lean forward from your hips and hold for a moment.**

3. **Relax your head and neck as you start rolling up your back and spine one vertebra at a time (see Figure 5-11b).**

4. **Finish the movement by rolling your shoulders back and down.**

Complete this exercise two or three times.

A few do's and don'ts for this exercise:

✔ *Do* roll up slowly, one vertebra at a time.

✔ *Don't* tense up your shoulders. Keep them relaxed and pressed down during this exercise.

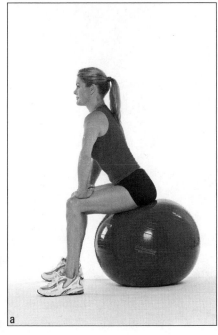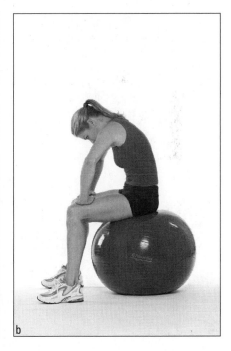

Figure 5-11:
Back
roll-up.

a

b

Chapter 6

A Swimmer's Body: Shoulders and Upper Back

....

In This Chapter

▶ Trying some shoulder and upper back exercises

▶ Building a broader and stronger you

....

*I*f you've ever watched a swim meet or the summer Olympics, you've probably noticed how amazingly fit these athletes are. One secret to looking slimmer is to define and tone your upper back and shoulders. It's definitely a smoke-and-mirrors trick that actually makes the waist appear smaller! It also draws attention upward; in fact, strong shoulders and a well-defined upper back are the first things people notice when you start getting in shape.

The exercises in this chapter introduce you to using the ball as a base while you work on the shoulders and upper back to achieve a swimmer's physique. I recommend starting your workout on the ball with this chapter because it follows the natural progression of working the body from the top to the bottom. If you're new to working out, try two of the four exercises in this chapter just to get acquainted with using the exercise ball. If you're ready for a challenge, do all four exercises in the prescribed order, and you'll also get a great abdominal workout from all the contracting you have to do just to keep your balance on the ball.

For now, you may want to try using only the resistance of your body rather than hand weights. When you begin feeling stable on the ball, feel free to add 3- to 5-pound hand weights for the exercises that incorporate weights.

Repetitions, repetitions, repetitions . . .

How many repetitions should I do? How many sets? What's the right amount for me?

All good questions, and the answers depend on the individual. Whether you do 10, 12, or 15 repetitions, the perfect amount is whatever feels right for you. The only reason to use repetitions is to keep track of your progress as you go. If I do 12 repetitions the first time I do an exercise,

then I can tell I'm getting stronger and better when 15 seems easy.

Make sure that you rest between sets. Resting gives the body a chance to refuel for the next set. Working on the ball is more about increasing endurance than using a lot of resistance, so keep your exercise simple — quality over quantity is a good way to go.

Seated Shoulder Press

This exercise is excellent for building upper body strength. I find that it really strengthens the muscles that come into play when I'm carrying my daughter around on my shoulders.

To do this exercise, follow these steps:

1. **Sit on the ball with your feet firmly planted on the ground. Keep your feet a little wider than hip-distance apart.**

2. **Place your arms at shoulder level with 3- to 5-pound weights in your hands, preparing for press-ups.**

3. **Press the weights upward and toward each other, touching them together at the very top. Make sure your palms are facing out and your arms are fully extended (see Figure 6-1).**

4. **Slowly bring your arms back down to starting position while tightening your abdominal muscles.**

Complete two sets of 12 repetitions.

A couple of do's and don'ts for this exercise:

✔ *Do* pinch your shoulder blades together by drawing your elbows back slightly at the beginning and end of the exercise.

✔ *Don't* let your shoulders tense up and float up to your ears as you do the workout.

What does the ball have to do with working my upper body?

You may be wondering why I recommend doing these back and shoulder exercises while sitting on a ball rather than standing or sitting in a chair. What connection does the ball have to your upper body? Well, you can certainly work your upper body without using a ball, but when you use a ball, you get a better, much more intense overall workout. How? The natural shape of the ball requires you to balance yourself on it, which gives you a more intense workout that's like no other. In addition, strengthening the core of your body and bringing awareness to the abdominal area are other great advantages to using an exercise ball in your fitness program as opposed to standing or sitting in a chair.

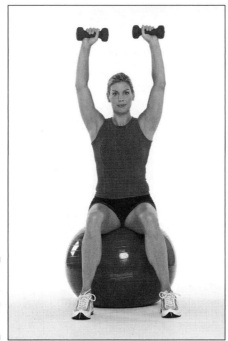

Figure 6-1:
Seated
shoulder
press.

Seated Lateral Arm Raise

Lateral arm raises really work the top of your shoulders, giving them great definition and shape. This exercise really helps with lifting groceries.

This exercise isn't as easy as it looks. You may want to start with just one set and work your way up as you go. To do this exercise, follow these steps:

1. **Start seated on the ball with your feet firmly placed on the ground, keeping them a little wider than hip-distance apart.**

   The setup is the same as the seated arm press.

2. **Place weights in your hands at your sides and bend your elbows to 90 degrees, as Figure 6-2a shows.**

   Keep your elbows firmly at your waist with your palms facing each other.

3. **Raise your arms out sideways, stopping at shoulder level (see Figure 6-2b).**

   Keep your hands and weights even with your elbows.

4. **Bring your arms back down to the starting position while tightening your abdominal muscles.**

   Elbows remain at your side until you begin the second repetition.

Figure 6-2:
Seated
lateral
arm raise.

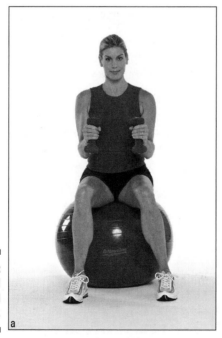
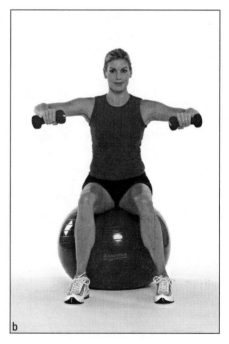

Complete two sets of 12 repetitions or start with one set of 15 repetitions for now.

A few do's and don'ts for this exercise:

✔ *Do* keep your back straight and lifted during this exercise.

✔ *Do* keep your neck and shoulders relaxed.

✔ *Don't* let your elbows go above your shoulders.

Seated Rows

Seated rows are a great way to work your upper back because they require a lot of control when doing them on the ball. This exercise also helps you maintain perfect posture. The forward and back motion is the same movement you use when you row a boat — hence, the name "row"!

To do this exercise, follow these steps:

1. **Sit on the ball with your feet firmly planted on the ground, keeping them a little wider than hip-distance apart.**

   The setup is the same as the lateral arm raise and the seated arm press.

2. **Place your weights in your hands with your palms facing up.**

   Keep your elbows firmly at your sides with your forearms at a 90-degree angle.

3. **Move your arms and weights directly out in front of you until you reach your knees (see Figure 6-3a).**

   As you perform this exercise, be sure not to reach too far forward with your arms. Doing so may cause you to lose your balance on the ball.

4. **Pull your arms back in toward you, bringing your elbows even with your waist (refer to Figure 6-3b).**

Complete two sets of 12 repetitions.

A few do's and don'ts for this exercise:

✔ *Do* keep your feet planted firmly on the ground as you extend your arms.

✔ *Do* keep your shoulders pressed down as you extend your arms.

✔ *Don't* use weights during this exercise if they make stabilizing the ball too challenging.

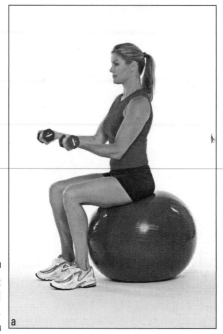 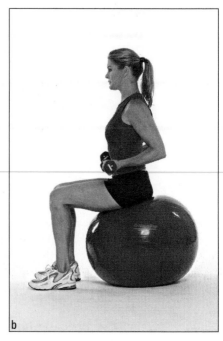

Figure 6-3:
Seated
rows.

a   b

Ball Lift with a Twist

The ball lift with a twist is similar to the "bob and weave" you may see boxers do, except this movement is more difficult when done on the ball. After using hand weights for the previous exercises, moving your shoulders a little from side to side feels good.

To do this exercise, follow these easy steps:

1. **Lie with your back on the ball and keep your feet planted firmly in front of you.**

   Make sure you have your heels directly below your knees. Your shoulders don't touch the ball, so they're free to move from side to side.

2. **Bring your arms to your chest and rest your chin on your hands (see Figure 6-4a).**

3. **Starting with your right shoulder, contract your abdominal muscles as you slowly lift and turn your body toward your left hip (see Figure 6-4b).**

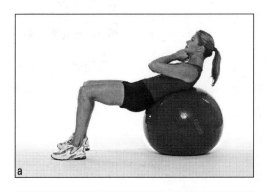

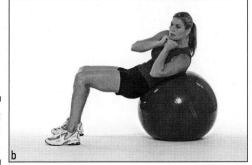

Figure 6-4:
Ball lift with
a twist.

4. **Stay lifted for a moment, and then slowly lower your body to the starting position.**

5. **Slowly lift your left shoulder as you contract your abdominal muscles and turn your body toward your right hip.**

Continue alternating your right- and left-side lifts for two sets of 12 repetitions — resting in between, of course!

A few do's and don'ts to keep in mind:

✔ *Do* exhale before you contract your abdominal muscles and lift.

✔ *Do* rest your chin on your hands for support.

✔ *Don't* rush through this exercise. Take a moment to pause at the top of the lift.

Chapter 7

Shapely, Sexy Arms

• •

In This Chapter

▶ Building stronger biceps using ball exercises

▶ Strengthening the triceps using ball exercises

▶ Performing forearm exercises on the ball

• •

*B*ecause muscle tone is a good indicator of overall fitness, I tell my clients that the best way to tell whether or not someone is in shape is to look at their arms. For women, maintaining muscle in the arms can be difficult because we lose muscle tone as we age. Add to that the fact that many different muscle groups make up the arms, so you need to work all the groups to keep your arms in shape. Even with all the lifting, pulling, and picking up you do throughout the day, you still need to work your arms to keep them beautifully toned.

In this chapter, I cover all three muscle groups of the arm — the biceps, the triceps, and the forearms. The exercises I include here make a well-balanced workout that will keep you looking fit and provide you with a sleek upper body.

Warm muscles work better

Getting your heart rate up before you lift weights is essential because warming up your muscles and tendons increases your muscle *elasticity* (muscle length and its ability to stretch with heat), which enables you to handle heavier weights. Increasing your heart rate also gives you the endurance you need for a longer workout.

You need only about five to ten minutes to increase your heart rate. Taking a spin on a bike or a short jog on the treadmill does the trick. Jumping rope for a few minutes is also a good warm-up because it definitely gets your heart pumping in no time. Plus, doing cardio before you strength train actually helps you burn more calories — and nothing's wrong with that!

Another good way to warm-up your body and have a little fun is by using the ball. Chapter 5 of this book shows you some great warm-up exercises that you can do with the ball — lifting it over your head, sitting on it, and even bouncing on it. To warm up your body properly before heading out the door to do any kind of sport, give the ball a chance! You may find you like the warm-up so much that you grab some hand weights and head right into Chapter 6 to work your shoulders and upper back.

Pump It Up!

Muscles! Men love them. Look at any bodybuilding competition, and the first muscles they flex are their arms.

I always like to know which muscle I'm working during a workout so I can visualize it getting bigger and stronger. Think about the body part that you're exercising so you can make a concentrated effort to flex it, contract it, or whatever you're trying to accomplish with it. Because many different muscles make up the arm, here's a brief overview of the muscles you work on in this chapter:

- ✔ **Biceps muscles:** The *biceps* start at the top of the shoulder joint and run down into the forearm. When you pull or push the ball, you use the biceps. The biceps are primarily responsible for bending your arms.

- ✔ **Triceps muscles:** The *triceps* are a little more complicated. They consist of three different muscles that run along the backs of your arms. The triceps are responsible for bending your elbows. Anytime you press something down and away from you, you use the triceps.

- ✔ **Forearm muscles:** The *forearms,* or lower arms, run from your elbow down to your wrist. These muscles often get neglected because many people know that the forearms get some exercise by working the biceps and triceps. Forearms are the muscles that boxers rely on the most because they give the hand the strength it needs to punch.

- ✔ **Shoulder muscles:** Finally, the *shoulder muscles* tie all these muscles together, so to speak. The shoulder muscle is made up of three muscles known as the *anterior, medial,* and *posterior deltoids;* together these muscles are called the *deltoids* or just the "delts." The delts help rotate your arm and raise it up and down and front to back. Anytime you raise your arms over your head, you work or use your shoulder muscles.

Sports-specific exercises

Did you ever wonder what sports-specific exercises were? I did, and now I know: They're exercises you can use to train a specific body part you use for a particular sport. Hence, the name "sports-specific exercises."

For the arms, some sports-specific training include racquet sports, swimming, gymnastics,

and weightlifting. Boxing is another sport that uses the arms and all kinds of interesting techniques to train them. Push-ups, jump rope, and shadowboxing are just a few exercises a boxer can use to stay strong, and all these exercises are considered sports-specific exercises.

Working the Biceps

Unlike the leg muscles, the biceps are a small muscle group, so you want to avoid overtraining them. You don't have to do too many repetitions to give them the sculpted look you're going for.

The following exercises use the ball as a base for sitting rather than as a weight bench. Using the ball challenges your balance and coordination, especially when you're working with weights. I suggest starting out with 3- to 5-pound hand weights; when you can comfortably do this workout two to three times a week, then work up to heavier dumbbells.

Biceps curls

To do the biceps curl, you need 3- to 5-pound weights. As you gain confidence and precision on the ball, use heavier dumbbells. The instability of the ball adds a new aspect of balancing to the biceps curl, making it more challenging.

To do this exercise, follow these steps:

1. **Sit on the ball with your feet shoulder-width apart. Hold your weights down by your sides with your palms facing inward.**

2. **Pull in your abdominal muscles as you slowly bring your weights toward your shoulders (see Figure 7-1).**

   Your palms will be facing your shoulder.

   As you curl the weights toward your shoulders, concentrate on the biceps muscles. Doing so helps you isolate the movement and focus on the muscle that you're working.

3. **Hold for a few beats and then release the weights back down to your sides.**

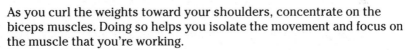

Complete two sets of 10 to 15 repetitions.

Here are a couple of do's and don'ts for this exercise:

- ✔ *Do* keep a straight spine while lifting the weights to your shoulders.
- ✔ *Do* lower the weights slowly back down to the starting position.
- ✔ *Don't* jerk the weights up to your shoulders; instead, use a small controlled movement.

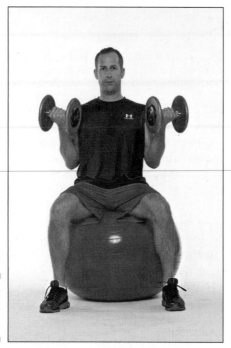

Figure 7-1:
Biceps
curls.

Alternating biceps curls

When doing alternating biceps curls, you may experience a subtle shifting of your weight on the ball, so concentrate on maintaining your balance throughout this exercise.

Beginners need 3- to 5-pound weights. Advanced men and women can use heavier dumbbells.

To do this exercise, follow these steps:

1. **Sit on the ball with your feet shoulder-width apart. Hold your weights down by your sides with your palms facing inward.**

2. **Pull in the abdominal muscles as you slowly bring your right weight toward your right shoulder (see Figure 7-2).**

   Your palm will face inward toward the shoulder.

3. **Hold for a few beats and then release the weight back down to your right side; repeat with your other arm.**

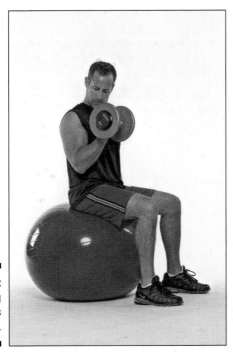

Figure 7-2:
Alternating
biceps
curls.

Complete two sets of ten repetitions.

A few do's and don'ts for this exercise:

- ✔ *Do* concentrate on your biceps muscles as you do this exercise.
- ✔ *Do* contract your abs before lifting the weight to your shoulder.
- ✔ *Don't* jerk the weight up to your shoulder; instead, use a slow and controlled movement.

Biceps curls with wall squat

The biceps curls with wall squat combines upper body strengthening with lower body toning. This exercise is great for targeting both areas at the same time.

Start out using 3- to 5-pound weights in each hand to maintain proper balance while doing this exercise. To increase the challenge, increase the weight and repetitions, as you feel more comfortable.

To do this exercise, follow these steps:

1. **Holding the weights in your hands, position the ball behind your back. Lower yourself into a seated squat position, keeping your hands down by your sides (see Figure 7-3a).**

2. **Stand up slowly, straightening yourself up out of the squat position as you bend your right elbow and curl the weight toward your shoulder (see Figure 7-3b).**

3. **Slowly squat back down as you lower the weights and straighten your elbow.**

4. **Repeat curling your left arm.**

Complete two sets of 10 to 15 repetitions.

A few do's and don'ts for this exercise:

✔ *Do* keep your back pressed into the ball as you straighten up into a standing position.

✔ *Do* straighten the arms fully after each biceps curl to get the full benefit of this exercise.

✔ *Don't* lean sideways during this exercise. Stand tall and straight, keeping the ball steady.

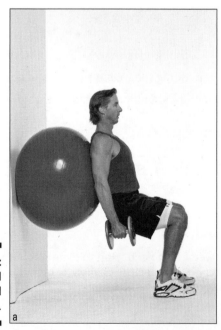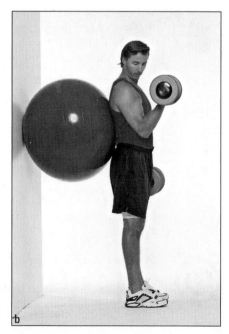

Figure 7-3: Biceps curl with wall squat.

a

b

Toning the Triceps

The triceps muscles are made up of three different muscles located along the back of your arms. The biceps muscles work in opposition to the triceps, so working both muscle groups is important in order to achieve balance and to keep the entire arm strong.

For these triceps exercises, you can do them with or without weights on the ball. I like doing the following exercises in this order, simply because you start out sitting on the ball and end standing.

After performing these moves, I recommend doing the triceps stretch shown in Chapter 14 to relieve any tightness that you may have built up in your muscles.

Seated triceps press

The triceps press works the triceps (the back of the arms). Like with the biceps curls, this exercise is more challenging when you do it on the ball because you need to maintain your balance.

If you have a neck or shoulder injury, always check with your doctor first to see which exercises are appropriate for you.

Beginners need one 3- to 5-pound weight. Advanced ball users can use a heavier dumbbell.

To do this exercise, follow these steps:

1. **Sit on the ball with your feet shoulder-width apart. Hold the weight in both hands behind your head (as Figure 7-4a shows).**

   Keep elbows close to your forehead.

2. **Straighten your elbows, pressing the weight toward the ceiling (see Figure 7-4b).**

3. **Bend your elbows to slowly lower the weight back down behind your neck.**

Complete two sets of ten repetitions.

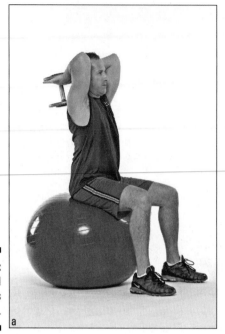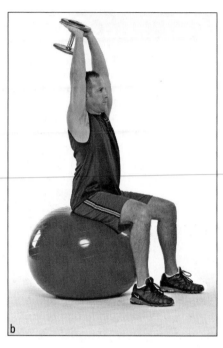

Figure 7-4:
Seated
triceps
press.

a | b

A couple of do's and don'ts for this exercise:

- *Do* hold the weight in both hands as you press up.

- *Don't* let your head and neck tilt forward during this exercise. Stare straight ahead and keep your neck long.

Triceps kickbacks

To end the triceps series, here are triceps kickbacks that you can do using the ball for support. The entire forearm gets a good workout with this exercise, especially if you increase the weight.

To do this exercise, follow these steps:

1. **Stand with your right hand and right knee firmly placed on the ball as you bring your torso even or parallel to the floor.**

   Your left knee will be slightly bent.

2. **Holding your weight in your left hand, keep your elbow bent at a 90-degree angle (as Figure 7-5a shows).**

3. **Using only your forearm, extend your arm behind you until the elbow is straight (see Figure 7-5b).**

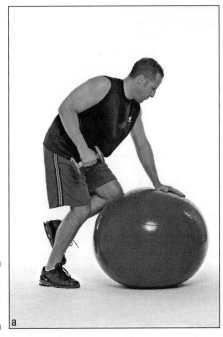 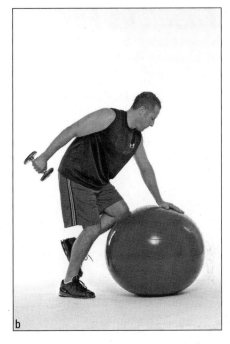

Figure 7-5:
Triceps
kickbacks.

4. **Hold your arm back for a few seconds and then return it to starting position.**

Complete ten repetitions and repeat using the opposite arm.

A couple of do's and don'ts for this exercise:

✔ *Do* keep your arm close to your side while performing this exercise.

✔ *Don't* arch your back. Keep it straight and long as you lift your forearm behind you.

✔ *Don't* let your head drop down.

Always lead with your hips, not your shoulders

Always keep your shoulders in line with your hips during any kind of twisting movement to avoid injury. Twisting can lead to serious back injuries because when you move the shoulders first, the hips stay behind. Next time you need to pick something up or look behind you, move the hips first so your shoulders move in unison.

Fabulous Forearms

The following exercises are classic weight-lifting exercises or bodybuilding techniques that I've adapted for use on the ball. However, when you perform an exercise on a chair or weight bench, you don't activate the stabilizing muscles that are so important for abdominal strength, good posture, and balance.

Seated hammer curls and reverse wrist curls work the entire forearm, biceps, and the wrists. Having strong wrists is especially important for making the little and big tasks of lifting throughout the day easier.

Seated hammer curls

Seated hammer curls help develop good biceps and forearms. Don't be afraid to challenge yourself by increasing the weight as you go along to possibly a 15-pound or heavier dumbbell.

To do this exercise, follow these steps:

1. **Sit tall on the ball with your feet hip-distance apart. Hold your weights in your hands with palms facing toward each other and your arms down by your sides (as Figure 7-6a shows).**

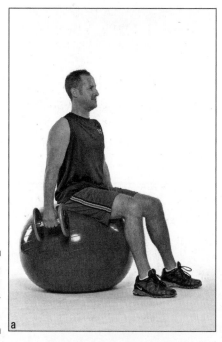 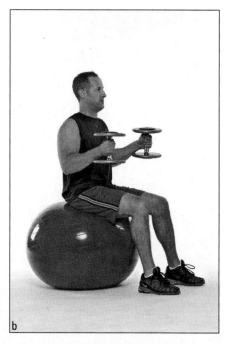

Figure 7-6: Seated hammer curls.

2. **Bend your elbows as you bring your weights toward your shoulders (see Figure 7-6b), keeping your abdominal muscles tight.**

   Be careful not to touch your shoulders with the weights.

3. **Slowly lower your weights back down, keeping tension on your biceps throughout the movement.**

Complete two sets of 10 to 15 repetitions.

A few do's and don'ts for this exercise:

- ✔ *Do* keep your feet firmly planted on the floor to keep the ball from moving.
- ✔ *Do* keep the elbows from moving back and forth during this exercise.
- ✔ *Don't* release the weights back down too fast. Use a slow and controlled movement throughout this exercise.

Seated reverse wrist curl

The reverse wrist curl builds up the muscles in the wrist. This exercise will eventually help you lift more weight when you're exercising your arms. For this exercise, you need 3- to 5-pound weights.

To do this exercise, follow these steps:

1. **Sit tall on the ball with your feet shoulder-width apart. Place your forearms on your thighs while holding a weight in each hand with your palms facing down.**

   Be sure to let your wrists hang over your knees.

2. **Bending at the wrists, lower the weights as far as possible, curling the wrists downward (see Figure 7-7a).**

3. **Lift the weights as high as you can to reverse the motion (as Figure 7-7b shows).**

Complete two sets of ten repetitions.

A few do's and don'ts for this exercise:

- ✔ *Do* keep your forearms pressed to your thighs.
- ✔ *Do* keep a tight hold on the weights as you curl your wrists.
- ✔ *Don't* lean too far forward on the ball when hanging your wrists over your knees.
- ✔ *Don't* allow your back to arch.

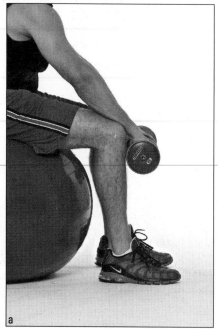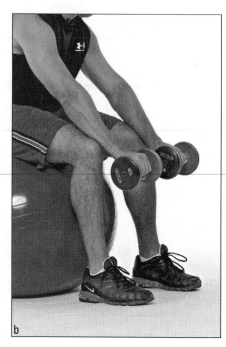

Figure 7-7:
Reverse
wrist curls.

Standing upright rows

This exercise works the entire arm and shoulder. Maintaining proper form throughout this exercise as you balance your knee on the ball is important.

To do this exercise, follow these steps:

1. **Place your right knee on the ball, keeping your upper torso almost parallel to the floor.**

2. **Balance yourself by keeping your left hand on the ball and holding your weight in your right hand at your side (see Figure 7-8a).**

3. **Pull your weight up with a rowing motion as your elbow pulls back past your rib cage (as Figure 7-8b shows).**

4. **Hold for a few seconds and then release your weight down to your side.**

Complete ten repetitions then switch sides and repeat.

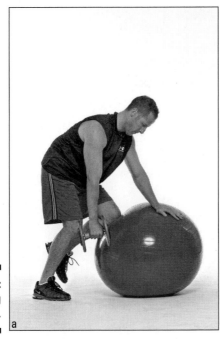
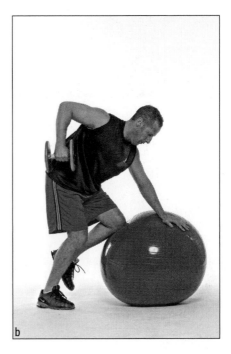

Figure 7-8:
Standing
rows.

A couple of do's and don'ts for this exercise:

✔ *Do* pull your elbow back as far as you can.

✔ *Don't* lift your head up, which causes your back to arch. Keep a long, straight spine during this exercise.

Chapter 8

Walking Tall: Chest, Abdominals, and Lower Back

*T*he *core* is a virtual powerhouse of strength located in the midsection of your body. Basically, your core includes everything between your ribs and your hips. In this chapter, I combine the best abdominal, chest, and lower back exercises to work your entire core.

I would say that the "no pain, no gain" expression applies best to this chapter. When you do the following exercises, I'm sure you'll discover strength that you never knew you had.

To get in the right frame of mind and to prepare your muscles and joints for the following exercises, try the warm-up in Chapter 5. Not only does it encourage circulation to your heart and lungs, but it also reduces the risk of injury.

Like with any new exercise program, consult your doctor before beginning. Never attempt any exercise that you're not sure of or that causes you pain in any way.

Man from horse!

If you visualize yourself with an invisible cord running from your chest up to the sky or a tree, you'll know why I call this section "Man from horse!" My dance teacher made this reference over and over in ballet class, and after I saw the movie starring Richard Harris, I got it. In case you haven't seen the movie, it features Richard Harris's character being strung up by his chest bone, or sternum, to a tree. Ouch! Of course my dance teacher referenced the movie because we were all slouching, and she was trying to make a point — the importance of good posture.

Slouching is a habit that's easy to fall into without even noticing. When I'm working at the computer, I always find myself slouching. Just recently I broke myself of this habit by replacing my chair with an exercise ball. It's amazing how sitting on something like a ball improves your posture within seconds! Sitting on the ball instead of a chair forces you to use the stabilizer muscles of the body and helps you develop strong balance. Sitting on the ball also makes you contract your abdominal muscles to steady yourself — it's an added benefit.

To replace your chair at work or at home with the ball, first make sure that the ball gives you the desired height and firmness you need. The desired height is when your thighs are parallel to the floor. The desired firmness is when the ball isn't too filled with air but has a slight give to it when you sit on it. In other words, when your butt makes a small indentation on the ball when you sit on it.

Lengthening Your Spine

As you move throughout the day, you use the muscles along your spine called the *multifidus muscles*. Bending down, picking things up, and twisting are all activities that use these muscles to protect the spinal cord. If you forget to strengthen the spine and back muscles, all your other activities suffer and your body weakens.

Many chiropractors and doctors use the lower back exercises in this chapter to keep the spine long and flexible. When you're in the *prone position* (lying face down) on the ball, you use all your muscles to support your body and to help build a stronger lower back.

After you complete the lower back exercises, I suggest trying the *back stretch* that I include in Chapter 14 or simply lying over the ball to stretch out your spine. My 3-year-old loves doing that exercise, and I hope you do, too!

Chest Workout

Many of the exercises in this section use your own body weight to build and strengthen the pecs, delts, and lats — otherwise known as the chest, shoulder, and upper back muscles.

The wall push-ups and floor push-ups both work the muscles in front of the chest, whereas the flies and lat pullovers concentrate on the muscles along the sides and the back of the body. In combination, the following exercises make for a complete and challenging workout.

Floor push-ups with the ball

Floor push-ups on the ball target your chest muscles along with your abdominal muscles and butt to keep you steady on the ball.

TIP

Keeping your lower legs or shins on the ball helps you balance yourself during the push-up.

To do this exercise, follow these steps:

1. **Lie with your belly on the ball and walk your hands forward until the ball rests under your legs (as Figure 8-1a).**

   Make sure that you keep your hands directly below your shoulders.

2. **Lower your upper body toward the floor, bending the elbows out to the sides (see Figure 8-1b).**

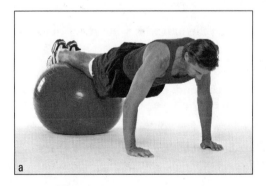

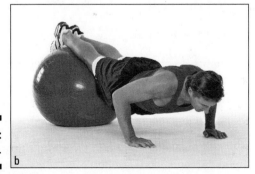

Figure 8-1:
Push-ups.

3. **Straighten your elbows and exhale as you press back up into starting position.**

Complete ten repetitions.

A couple of do's and don'ts for this exercise:

✔ *Do* keep your abdominal muscles tight to help you maintain your balance.

✔ *Do* use proper breathing, inhaling as you slowly lower your body down and exhaling as you press your body back up.

✔ *Don't* arch your back. Keep it straight and in line with your head and the rest of your body.

Chest press with bridge

The chest press with a bridge combines two great exercises — the bridge and the chest press — to work the pectoral, hips, and butt muscles.

Keep your hips pressed up toward the ceiling during this exercise. Any sagging or arching in your lower back can place strain on your back muscles.

To do this exercise, follow these steps:

1. **Rest your upper back on the ball with your knees bent at a 90-degree angle.**

   Make sure that your knees are stacked over your ankles.

2. **Holding a weight in each hand, extend your arms toward the ceiling, placing the weights directly above your chest (as Figure 8-2 shows).**

   Your palms will face forward as you press your weights up.

3. **Lower your weights back down by bending your elbows back in toward your body.**

Complete two sets of 10 to 15 repetitions.

A couple of do's and don'ts for this exercise:

✔ *Do* slowly press the weights up above your head feeling your chest muscles contract.

✔ *Don't* forget to tighten your abdominal muscles to support your back.

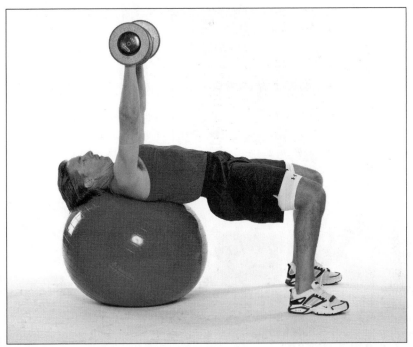

Figure 8-2:
Chest press
with bridge.

Flys on the ball

This exercise is a lot harder than the traditional fly exercises you're probably used to doing on a weight bench. Not only do you rest your upper back on the ball, but you also use your abs and hips to keep the ball from rolling out from under you.

To do this exercise, follow these steps:

1. **Lie with your upper back on the ball and bend your knees at a 90-degree angle.**

2. **Holding the weights in your hands, extend your arms straight up toward the ceiling and above your chest (see Figure 8-3a).**

3. **With your palms facing each other, slowly lower your arms out sideways (see Figure 8-3b).**

   Your elbows will be slightly bent when you open them out to the side.

4. **Using your chest muscles, bring the weights back up toward the ceiling to the starting position.**

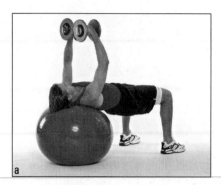

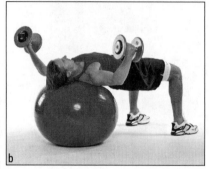

Figure 8-3: Flies on the ball.

Complete two sets of 10 to 15 repetitions.

A few do's and don'ts for this exercise:

- ✔ *Do* tighten your butt muscles to support your back and pelvis.
- ✔ *Do* keep your weights directly above your chest when you lift them overhead.
- ✔ *Don't* open your arms so wide that you arch your back.
- ✔ *Don't* forget to perform this exercise slowly, using controlled movements throughout.

Lat pullover on the ball

Working the lats (or *latissimus dorsi*) gives you a sculpted upper back and well-defined shoulders. Building up the lats also makes your waist appear smaller.

When you combine this exercise with the ball, you get the added benefits of working the butt and the hips as you press up into the classic bridge position. For this exercise, you need a 3- to 5-pound weight.

To do this exercise, follow these steps:

1. **Lie with your upper back on the ball and keep your knees bent at a 90-degree angle.**

2. **Holding the weight in your hands, extend your arms straight above your chest toward the ceiling.**

3. **Slowly lower the weight behind your head, slightly bending your elbows (see Figure 8-4a).**

   Don't let the weight drop too far below your head. To avoid this problem, keep your elbows soft and slightly bent.

4. **Raise the weight and your arms back toward the ceiling and above your chest (as Figure 8-4b shows).**

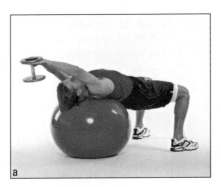

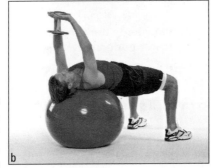

Figure 8-4:
Lat pullover
on the ball.

Complete two sets of ten repetitions.

A few do's and don'ts for this exercise:

✔ *Do* avoid arching your back.

✔ *Do* keep your feet shoulder-width apart to help maintain your balance.

✔ *Don't* forget to keep a tight grip on the weight as you raise your arms above and behind your head.

Lower Back

Working the lower back on the exercise ball offers you a better alternative to the traditional methods of exercising the back because it provides support for the pelvis and lumbar spine at the same time.

By supporting the hips, the ball allows the lower body to go through a greater range of movements, enhancing the strengthening benefits to the back muscles and spine. Because of the *prone* (or face down) position used throughout this series of exercises, the following exercises support and strengthen the upper back as well as the lower back muscles.

Prone on the ball

Lying prone on the ball is great position for strengthening all the muscles along the spine. Lying prone on the ball also gives you good posture and balance.

To do this exercise, follow these steps:

1. **Kneeling behind the ball, roll your body forward and to the other side so the ball supports your lower abdominal muscles.**

   The ball will be under your hips, and your hands will rest on the floor in front of you.

2. **Slowly raise your chest, creating a straight line from your shoulders to your feet (see Figure 8-5).**

3. **Hold up your chest by using your back muscles for a few seconds; then relax your chest back onto the ball.**

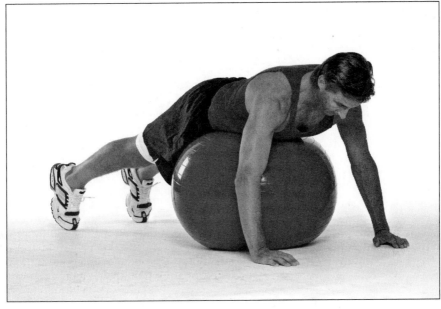

Figure 8-5:
Prone
position
on the ball.

Stay in this position for a few minutes, extending and relaxing. This move-ment gives you a feel for how you'll need to use the lower back muscles to stabilize yourself throughout this series of exercises.

A couple of do's and don'ts for this exercise:

✔ *Do* keep your feet close together to maintain your balance on the ball.

✔ *Don't* balance on your toes. Make sure that you're on the balls of your feet for support.

Prone leg raises

Prone leg raises test your strength and balance by using an alternating lifting motion for the lower body and a balancing movement for the upper body.

To do this exercise, follow these steps:

1. **Lie prone on the ball with your fingertips lightly touching the ground in front of you for support.**

2. **Keeping your body horizontal to the floor, raise one leg behind you to hip level (as Figure 8-6 shows).**

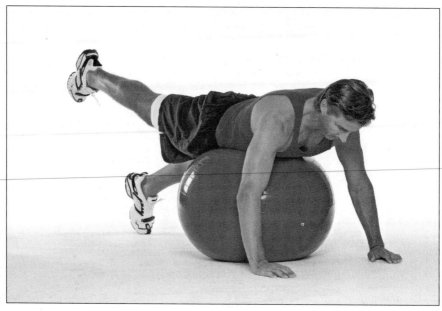

Figure 8-6:
Prone leg
raises.

The knee will be straight on the leg that's raised.

3. **Hold the position for a few seconds before lowering the leg down to starting position and raising the opposite leg.**

Complete two sets of ten kicks on each leg, resting in between sets.

A few do's and don'ts for this exercise:

✔ *Do* keep your leg straight when you extend it behind you, forming a straight line from your toes to your shoulders.

✔ *Do* keep your eyes looking straight down at the floor to avoid hyper-extending your neck.

✔ *Don't* forget to kick from the butt using your gluteal muscles.

Alternating arm and leg raises

This exercise can be quite challenging because as you raise your arms and legs, you need to stabilize yourself on the ball at the same time in order to keep your balance.

Before you begin, try finding your balance by lifting both hands off the floor. By doing this, having better balance throughout this exercise will be easier.

To do this exercise, follow these steps:

1. **Lie prone on the ball, resting your fingertips lightly on the floor in front of you.**

2. **Raise your right arm off the floor in front of you as you lift your left leg as far as hip level (see Figure 8-7a).**

3. **Lower your right arm back to the floor as you simultaneously lower your left leg.**

4. **Raise your left arm off the floor in front of you as you lift your right leg as far as hip level (see Figure 8-7b).**

5. **Lower your left arm back to the floor as you simultaneously lower your right leg.**

Continue alternating arm and leg raises. Complete two sets of ten repetitions, resting between sets.

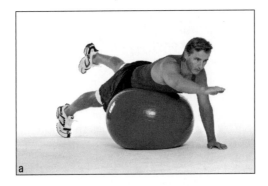

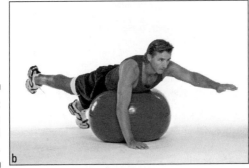

Figure 8-7:
Alternating
arm and
leg raises.

A few do's and don'ts for this exercise:

✔ *Do* keep your knees straight when you lift your leg behind you.

✔ *Do* use your butt to lift your leg, being sure to work from the gluteal muscles.

✔ *Don't* strain your neck. Keep your eyes looking straight down to the floor.

Amazing Abs!

The best way to get killer abs is by using the exercise ball because its round shape helps place extra emphasis on the abdominal muscles. Throughout these abdominal exercises, your body calls upon the stabilizing muscles (your core muscles) to support your weight on the ball, increasing the challenge and benefits.

Traditional abdominal crunches work the outer muscles known as the *rectus abdominus*. Working these muscles in conjunction with the deeper abdominal muscles called upon to stabilize your spine while using the ball is the best way to target the entire core of the body.

Abdominal curls

Perhaps the number-one exercise used on the ball is the abdominal curl. Harder than traditional curls and requiring more endurance, this abdominal exercise will be sure to kick your butt!

To do this exercise, follow these steps:

1. **Lie with the ball under your lower back and pelvis for support. Place your feet shoulder-width apart and keep your knees at a 90-degree angle.**

2. **With your hands behind your head and your elbows bent out to the sides, curl your body up halfway between a sitting and lying position (as Figure 8-8 shows).**

   Keep your tailbone pressed down on the ball.

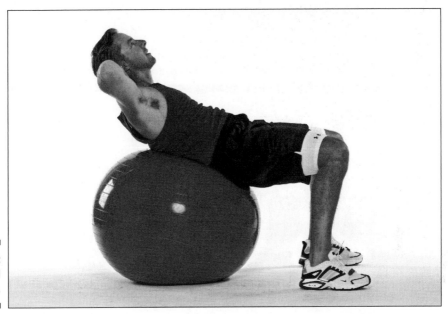

Figure 8-8:
Abdominal
curls.

3. Slowly roll back down onto the ball, one vertebrae at a time.

Complete two sets of 10 to 15 repetitions.

A few do's and don'ts for this exercise:

✔ *Do* draw your navel toward your spine when you contract your abdominal muscles to curl up.

✔ *Do* exhale as you lift up.

✔ *Do* curl up and roll back down one vertebrae at a time to keep from straining your back.

✔ *Don't* pull on your neck with your hands. Keep your gaze upward as you curl up to keep your neck in line with your spine.

Side crunch

The side crunch works the muscles that run along the waist otherwise known as the *obliques*. This exercise is great for men and women who want to define their waistlines and lose their love handles!

To do this exercise, follow these steps:

1. **Kneeling on the floor, position your left hip and side of your body against the ball as you place your left arm on the ball for support. Straighten your right leg out to the side and bring your right arm behind your head, so your hand is touching the back of your head (see Figure 8-9a).**

2. **Crunch up, bringing your right shoulder and elbow down toward your rib cage and right leg as you exhale (see Figure 8-9b).**

   Be sure to keep your left hip and side against the ball at all times to keep from slipping.

3. **Lower back down toward the ball as you slowly inhale.**

Complete ten side crunches before switching sides.

A few do's and don'ts for this exercise:

   ✔ *Do* keep the foot on your extended leg flat on the floor at all times for balance.

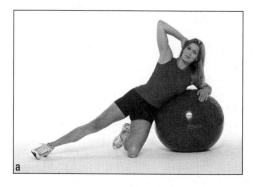

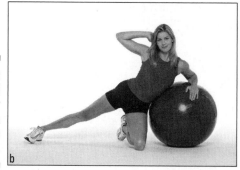

Figure 8-9:
Trim and tighten your waist with the side crunch.

✔ *Do* place your foot against a wall if you find yourself slipping.

✔ *Don't* forget to exhale as you crunch up, bringing your elbow down toward your knee.

Roll away

Perhaps the second-most popular exercise for working the abdominal muscles is the roll away. This exercise is a great way to target your abs from the inside out.

To do this exercise, follow these steps:

1. **Kneeling in front of the ball, place your hands on the ball at arm's length (see Figure 8-10a).**

2. **As you contract your abdominal muscles and tuck in your butt, roll the ball away from you slightly so that your forearms rest on the ball (see Figure 8-10b).**

3. **Keeping your butt tucked in and your back straight, hold this movement for a few seconds before you return to starting position.**

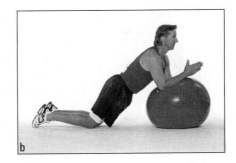

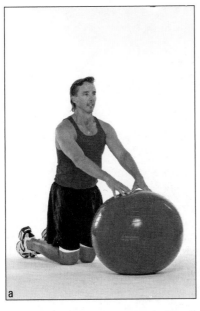

Figure 8-10: Roll away.

To increase the challenge, roll the ball away from you a little farther. You can also try rolling the ball slightly from side to side.

Complete one set of 15 repetitions.

A few do's and don'ts for this exercise:

- ✔ *Do* kneel on a cushion or mat if your knees start hurting.

- ✔ *Do* keep your back long and straight to keep it from arching.

- ✔ *Don't* hold the movement for a few seconds when the ball is rolled out in front of you if you find this exercise too challenging. Simply roll the ball out and back without holding in between.

Oblique twists

Because of the twisting motion in this exercise, your waist and your oblique muscles get a workout along with your abs.

To do this exercise, follow these easy steps:

1. **Lie with your back on the ball and your feet planted firmly out in front of you.**

   Make sure you have your heels directly below your knees.

   Your shoulders will not touch the ball, so they're free to move from side to side.

2. **Bring your arms to your chest and rest your chin on your hands (see Figure 8-11a).**

3. **Starting with your right shoulder, contract your abdominal muscles as you slowly lift and turn your body toward your left hip (see Figure 8-11b).**

4. **Keep your body lifted for a moment, and then slowly lower your body to the starting position.**

5. **Slowly lift your left shoulder as you contract your abdominal muscles and turn your body toward your right hip.**

Continue alternating your right and left side lifts for two sets of 12.

A few do's and don'ts to keep in mind:

- ✔ *Do* exhale before you contract your abdominal muscles and lift.

- ✔ *Do* rest your chin on your hands for support.

- ✔ *Don't* rush through this exercise. Take a moment to pause at the top of the lift.

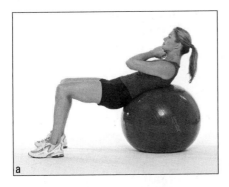

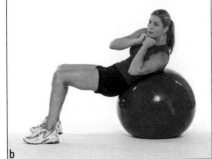

Figure 8-11:
Oblique
twist.

Abdominal crunch

Doing abdominal crunches with the ball places the emphasis not only on the abs but also on the legs, butt, and hips. By grasping the ball under your knees, the larger abdominal muscles, or outer abdominals, get used a lot more intensely during this exercise.

To do this exercise, follow these steps:

1. **Lying on the floor, rest your lower legs on the ball at a 90-degree angle (see Figure 8-12a).**

2. **As you tighten your abdominals, grasp the ball between your legs and pull toward you, lifting the ball from the floor.**

3. **With your hands on either side of your head, slowly lift your shoulders from the floor toward your knees (see Figure 8-12b).**

4. **Hold the lift for a few seconds and then slowly roll your shoulders back to the floor.**

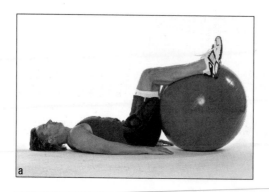

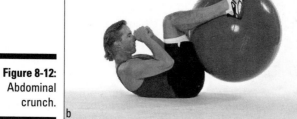

Figure 8-12:
Abdominal
crunch.

Complete ten repetitions.

A couple of do's and don'ts for this exercise:

- ✔ *Do* relax your neck as you curl up into a crunch.
- ✔ *Don't* forget to exhale as you curl up and inhale as you release back down.

Chapter 9

Booty Patrol: Working the Butt, Legs, and Hips

In This Chapter

▶ Working your lower half on the ball

▶ Getting a great butt

▶ Developing stronger legs

▶ Shaping up your hips

*N*ot since Jennifer Lopez came along has there been so much emphasis on having a more pronounced, shapelier butt. A firm butt that can fill out a bathing suit has suddenly caught the attention of the fashion world and the rest of us! The *Butt Blaster, Buns of Steel,* and my very own *Firm* video called *Abs, Hips and Thighs* all focus on one thing and one thing only: how to get a rounder tush.

As you age, excess weight tends to gravitate toward the lower half of the body. By now, most of you've probably discovered this phenomenon for yourself. For women, the extra pounds usually come from giving birth. For men, they usually sneak up from lack of exercise due to an old football injury or sitting around watching too much Monday Night Football.

Because of the large muscle groups that exist in the lower half of the body, you can work this area effectively and more efficiently than other areas. In this chapter, I include a killer workout for your glutes, legs, and hips. After you conquer this workout, try the upper body workouts in Chapters 6 and 7 for your arms, shoulders, chest, and upper back to even things out a bit.

Before you begin this workout, do five to ten minutes of cardio exercise. You can jump rope or take a brisk walk that starts at a slow pace and ends at a faster one.

Try doing some lower body stretching, too, to increase your flexibility and to help prepare your body by increasing core temperature before your workout (see Chapter 14, where you'll find the quad stretch, hamstring stretch, butt and back stretch, and gluteal stretch). I also suggest stretching after your workout to prevent any stiffness or soreness that may have accumulated in your lower back.

That Trouble Area: The Lower Half

Alright, here are the three main movements you'll be using to work your lower half in the following exercises: squeezing, stretching, and stepping.

Here's why doing the following exercises in this chapter will give you the "perfect ending":

- **Squeezing:** Your *glutes* are made up of three major muscles that work together to move your thigh away from your body or out to the side, to allow your leg to stretch out behind you, and to turn your leg in and out as needed. As you lift up your hips during the "butt lift," single leg bridge, leg circles, and hip flexion exercises, you squeeze (or contract) your glutes to create a shapelier derriere.

- **Stretching:** Your *hamstrings* and *quadriceps* are the muscles that make up the upper leg, and you need to stretch these muscles so they can gain strength and provide stability throughout the lower body. As you stretch out these muscles in your legs and butt in opposite directions for the hip extension exercise and in the prone leg raises, you increase the stretch in the gluteal muscles and the lower leg muscles, which creates a leaner lower body.

- **Stepping:** The *hip flexors* allow you to bend your hips and upper legs, and you use them when you step into a lunge or take one big step forward. As you do the wall lunge exercise or the wall squat, you use your hip flexors to control the movement and strengthen your hip joints as you maintain your body weight with your quadriceps and hamstrings or lower legs.

A Great Rear View

The following exercises may be a pain in the rear, but, ultimately, they'll pay off big time, giving you a leaner, toner lower body and a shapelier butt.

In Chapter 5, you find a good warm-up to get your circulation going (ball bounces) and to increase the flexibility in your hip joints before you begin the following workout. Walking is a good all-around exercise that can help alleviate built-up tension in the lower half of your body, so I strongly suggest adding it at the beginning or end of this workout.

Wall squat

By placing the ball between your body and the wall, a standard squat position becomes a much more difficult squat. This one is a great exercise you can do to literally work your butt off!

To do this exercise, follow these steps:

1. **Place the ball between the wall and your lower back, and walk your feet out slightly.**

2. **Lower your body into a squat position as you push your weight back into the ball (see Figure 9-1).**

   Hold this squat position for 5 seconds before straightening your legs and returning to starting position.

   Bend your knees at a 90-degree angle or as far as you feel comfortable.

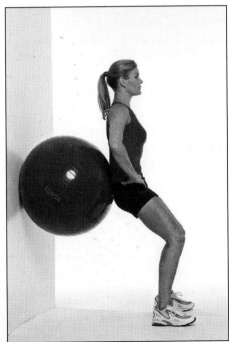

Figure 9-1:
Wall squat.

3. **Straighten your legs, keeping your weight over your heels to return to standing position.**

Complete 10 to 15 repetitions.

A couple of do's and don'ts for this exercise:

✔ *Do* keep your feet pointing straight forward as you lower down into a squatting position.

✔ *Don't* rush the movement.

✔ *Don't* let your knees roll out to the sides. Keep them in line with the rest of your body.

Wall lunge

This exercise combines a lunge with the ball, which adds resistance to increase the difficulty. The wall lunge strongly defines your butt and quadricep muscles.

To avoid placing strain on your knees, never extend them past your toes.

To do the wall lunge, follow these steps:

1. **With your feet hip-width apart, place the ball between the wall and your lower back or tailbone.**

2. **Step forward into a lunge position with one leg, bending your front knee at a 90-degree angle and keeping your back heel lifted (see Figure 9-2).**

As you lunge forward, be sure to keep your tailbone pressed into the ball to maintain your balance.

Hold the lunge position for 5 seconds.

3. **Use your butt and hamstring muscles to press yourself back up to standing position. Change legs and repeat the movement on the other side.**

Complete two sets of 10 to 15 repetitions.

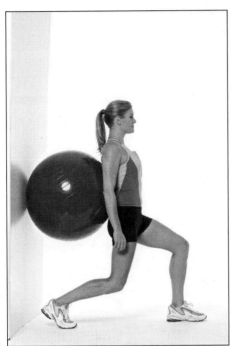

Figure 9-2:
Wall lunge.

A few do's and don'ts for this exercise:

✔ *Do* keep your back straight, your head up, and your chest lifted during this exercise.

✔ *Do* hold the lunge position for a few seconds before pressing back up to the standing position.

✔ *Don't* hyperextend your knee by letting it move beyond your toes.

Butt lifts

The butt lift is basically the bridge exercise (see Chapter 11) combined with an added press-up to increase the amount of weight you put on your hips and lower back.

As you lift your hips up, you need to keep your back from sagging or arching.

To do this exercise, follow these steps:

1. **Rest your head and shoulders on the ball and bend your knees at a 90-degree angle (see Figure 9-3a).**

   Make sure that you keep your knees stacked over your ankles.

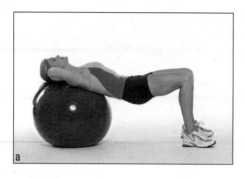

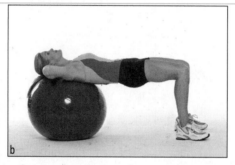

Figure 9-3:
Butt lifts.

> **2. Press your hips as high as possible toward the ceiling (see Figure 9-3b).**
>
> **3. Slowly lower your hips down to starting position.**

Complete 10 to 15 repetitions.

A few do's and don'ts for this exercise:

- ✔ *Do* rest the back of your head on the ball during this exercise.
- ✔ *Don't* let your hips and butt sink toward the ground. Keep your lower body tight and pressed up during this exercise.

Prone leg raises

This exercise helps you develop tighter buns and a longer leg line from all the reaching that you do as you lie with your stomach on the ball (otherwise known as the prone position; see Chapter 8). Prone leg raises also test your strength and balance because they require you to balance your upper body as you use an alternating lifting motion for your lower body.

To do this exercise, follow these steps:

1. **Lie prone over the ball with your fingertips lightly touching the ground in front of you for support.**

2. **Keeping your body horizontal to the floor, raise one leg behind you to hip level (as Figure 9-4 shows).**

   Your knee will be straight on the leg that's raised.

3. **Hold this pose for a few seconds before you lower your leg to starting position and raise your opposite leg.**

Complete two sets of ten raises on each leg, resting between sets.

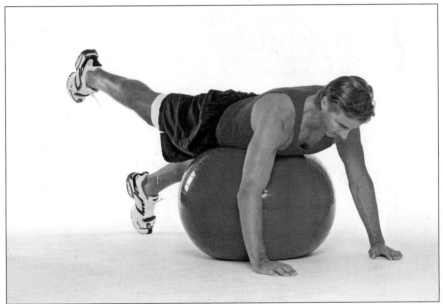

Figure 9-4:
Prone leg
raises.

A few do's and don'ts for this exercise:

✔ *Do* keep your eyes looking straight down at the floor to avoid hyperextending your neck.

✔ *Do* keep your leg straight when extending it behind you so that it forms a straight line from your toes to your shoulders.

✔ *Don't* forget to use your gluteal muscles to raise your leg.

Alternating arm and leg raises

This exercise is quite challenging because, as you raise your arm and legs simultaneously, you also need to stabilize yourself on the ball by really squeezing your glutes together.

Before you begin, find your balance by lying with your tummy on the ball and lifting both hands off the floor. This way you have better balance throughout the exercise.

To do this exercise, follow these steps:

1. **Lie face down on the ball, resting your fingertips lightly on the floor in front of you.**

2. **Raise your right arm off the floor in front of you as you lift your left leg as far as hip level (see Figure 9-5a).**

3. **Lower your right hand back to the floor as you simultaneously lower your left leg.**

4. **Raise your left arm off the floor in front of you as you lift your right leg as far as hip level (see Figure 9-5b).**

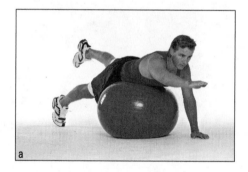

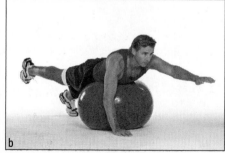

Figure 9-5:
Alternating
arm and
leg raises.

5. **Lower your left arm back to the floor as you simultaneously lower your right leg.**

6. **Continue alternating arm and leg raises.**

Complete two sets of ten repetitions, resting between sets.

A few do's and don'ts for this exercise:

- ✔ *Do* keep your knees straight when you lift your leg behind you.
- ✔ *Do* use your butt to lift your legs, being sure to work from the gluteal muscles.
- ✔ *Don't* strain your neck. Keep your eyes looking straight toward the floor.

Hot Legs!

Even if you don't like your hips or inherited a pear-shaped body, that doesn't mean you can't have great legs. Building strong hamstrings, toned quadriceps, and shapelier calf muscles will make you look and feel good enough to wear shorts all year round.

In the following exercises, you use the resistance of the floor combined with balancing your body weight on the ball to help you build stronger, leaner legs in no time.

Hamstring lift

The hamstring lift works your entire lower body, which includes your hips, lower back, and legs. Because you have to use your lower legs to control the movement of the ball, this exercise also challenges your calf muscles.

To do this exercise, follow these steps:

1. **Lie on the floor with your feet on top of the ball (see Figure 9-6a).**

    Place your arms on the floor alongside your body for support.

2. **Exhale as you raise your hips and pelvis toward the ceiling, pressing down into the ball with your feet to maintain your balance (see Figure 9-6b).**

3. **Inhale as you slowly lower your hips back down toward the floor.**

Complete ten repetitions.

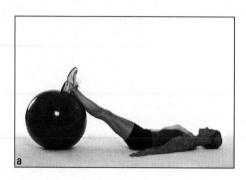

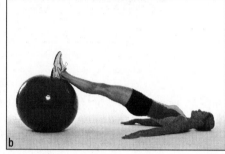

Figure 9-6:
Hamstring
lift.

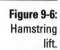

A few do's and don'ts for this exercise:

- ✔ *Do* keep your feet relaxed when they're resting on the ball.
- ✔ *Do* lift your hips straight up toward the ceiling hips and keep a straight back.
- ✔ *Don't* lift your chin. Keep it tucked into your chest.

Leg circles

The lifting motion the hips use in this exercise helps create shapelier legs and a tighter butt. By working the muscles in your upper legs and alongside your hips, you'll notice better buns in no time!

To do this exercise, follow these steps:

1. **As you lie on the floor, place your left leg on the ball and extend your right leg toward the ceiling (as Figure 9-7a shows).**

2. **Keeping your shoulders on the floor, lift your hips and extend your leg straight above you (see Figure 9-7b).**

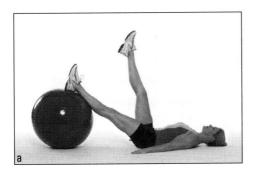

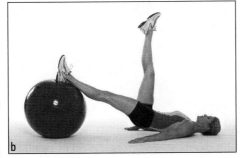

Figure 9-7:
Leg circles.

3. **Point your toe and use your leg to make five small circles to the right and then five small circles to the left.**

4. **Lower your leg back to the ball and return your hips to the floor.**

5. **Repeat this movement on the other side.**

Complete five sets on each side.

A few do's and don'ts for this exercise:

- ✔ *Do* keep your arms flat on the floor alongside your body for support.
- ✔ *Don't* forget to contract your abs before you lift your hips off the floor.
- ✔ *Don't* tense your neck and shoulders as you lift your leg off the ball.

Single-leg bridge

The single-leg bridge is a variation of the classic bridge exercise. But the single-leg bridge targets your hamstrings, quadriceps, and glutes, which provides you with a more toned lower half and leaner legs. The single-leg bridge uses only one leg to support the weight of your entire body, so your all-important core (abs and butt muscles) also gets a good workout.

To do this exercise, follow these steps:

1. **Sit tall on the ball and roll down slowly until only your shoulders touch the ball.**

2. **As you contract your abs, place your left leg across your right thigh (see Figure 9-8a).**

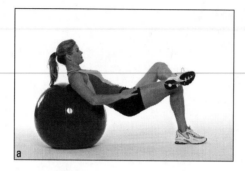

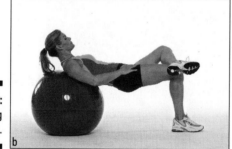

Figure 9-8:
Single-leg
bridge.

3. **Lift your hips toward the ceiling as you contract your butt muscles (see Figure 9-8b).**

   If you find the ball moving during this exercise, place it against the wall or a heavy piece of furniture.

4. **Pause for a moment and then lower your hips.**

Complete ten repetitions before you switch legs and repeat on the other side.

A couple of do's and don'ts for this exercise:

✔ *Do* keep your hands on your hips to help steady your body.

✔ *Don't* press your hips too high. Keep them even with your torso.

Work Those Hip Flexors

The hips can be tough to target and isolate; however, the following exercises do just that. By extending and flexing your hip joints, this trouble area (big hips and flabby thighs) will be problem-free in no time.

Hip extension

In this exercise, extending your leg behind you and placing your hips over the ball works both your butt and leg muscles to help support your body and help you stay lifted.

Because you kneel on the floor in this exercise, you may want to place a floor mat or towel under your knees for more comfort.

To do this exercise, follow these steps:

1. **Kneel with your chest on the ball and tighten your abdominal muscles.**

   Your hands will be resting on the ball for support.

2. **Extend your right leg and left arm slowly until they're opposite each other (as Figure 9-9 shows).**

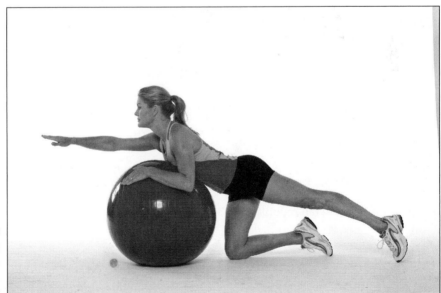

Figure 9-9:
Hip
extension.

Your right hand will still rest on the ball for support. Be sure you keep your back straight and in line with your arms and legs.

You should be able to draw an imaginary line down the center of your body.

3. **Point your toe and hold that pose for a few seconds before you return to your starting position.**

Complete five extensions on each side.

A couple of do's and don'ts for this exercise:

✔ *Do* keep your spine on the same plane or level with your raised arm and leg.

✔ *Don't* arch your back when you extend your arm and leg out over the ball.

Hip flexion

Your hips get a great workout with this exercise by pulling the ball into your body and resting your weight on the ball. As a result, you strengthen and tone your hips and your entire lower body.

Be sure you use your hips rather than your legs to pull in the ball.

To do this exercise, follow these steps:

1. **Lie with the ball under your stomach and roll forward until the ball rests under your shins (as Figure 9-10a shows).**

2. **Pull the ball in using your hips, and slowly bring your knees into your chest (see Figure 9-10b).**

   The top of your head will relax toward the floor and be in line with your spine.

3. **Hold this position for a few seconds and then slowly extend your legs back into the starting position.**

Complete ten repetitions.

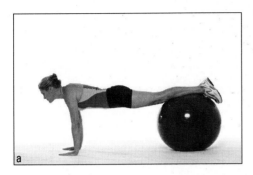

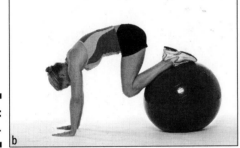

Figure 9-10:
Hip flexion.

A few do's and don'ts for this exercise:

✔ *Do* use your hips to roll the ball toward your chest.

✔ *Don't* arch your lower back at all during this exercise.

✔ *Don't* hyperextend your neck by looking up. Keep your gaze toward the floor.

Chapter 10

Cool It! Wrapping Up Your Workout with Easy Moves and Stretches

. . . .

In This Chapter

▶ Knowing why you need to cool down properly

▶ Cooling down using the ball

. . . .

Cooling down before you run out of a workout class or jump in the shower is important for several reasons. The most important reason to cool down is to reduce the risk of injuring yourself. I like comparing cooling down after a workout to cooking a turkey on Thanksgiving. (I'm aware of how odd this sounds, but hang in there.) The truth is, you can't serve your turkey as soon as you take it out of the oven without allowing the juices to flow back into the bird — unless you don't mind your turkey tasting like cardboard. When you exercise, you need time after working out to allow the blood to return to your muscles, heart, and lungs. If you don't cool your body down, you run the risk of fainting, pulling a muscle, or feeling just plain sore the next day.

In this chapter, I include exercises that slowly cool your body down, and I end with a few gentle stretches for your back and lower body. Also, be sure you hold each stretch for 10 to 15 seconds.

If you have the time, I recommend taking 10 to 15 minutes to cool down completely. One of the greatest things about taking the time to cool down is the feeling of deep relaxation that you feel when your workout's all over. Giving yourself this extra time at the end of your workout helps you concentrate and focus better on all the activities that lie ahead of you so you can have fun and stay relaxed!

If you're in a pinch or the total time of your workout consists of a half hour or less, cooling down for 5 to 10 minutes will do just fine. The general rule for cooling down is to allow yourself enough time at the end of your workout to return to breathing normally and to loosen any muscles that feel sore, tight, or cramped from your workout. Cooling down properly is also important because it encourages circulation back to the heart and lungs and lets your body return to its pre-exercise heart rate.

Cooling Down the Right Way

Whatever activity you choose to do for your workout, take the time to cool down properly because you enhance the benefits of your workout. You really feel yourself reducing your risk of injury as well as any soreness.

You can loosen up your muscles to reduce the risk of injury in many different ways after you've raised your heart rate. But no matter how you choose to do so, remember these two important points:

✔ Do it gradually.

✔ Use a very low intensity exercise.

One good way to cool down (that's convenient and fun) is walking. Of course, I don't mean just walking to your car after your workout. What I mean is walking 5 to 10 minutes at a slow pace to give your body the time it needs to recharge.

Another good way to cool down is to spend 3 to 5 minutes on a treadmill walking at a slow, comfortable pace (you want to make sure you keep your arms at your sides to keep them from swinging and increasing your heart rate).

Whatever form of light exercise you choose to do for your cool down, it should mimic some of the movements you used in your workout (if you were running, a light jog ending with a slow walking pace would work best). You should also include some deep breathing to help the blood flow back to your heart, lungs, and muscles to oxygenate your system.

After you've slowed down your heart rate, stretching is a great way to take your body's core temperature down and to increase your flexibility. You've probably seen a runner holding onto a lamppost to stretch out her calves or holding her ankle behind her to stretch out her hamstrings immediately after a run. Runners really know the importance of stretching immediately after a run to keep their bodies loose and flexible.

To minimize injury prior to exercising when your muscles are cold, you should limit pre-exercise stretches to no longer than 3 minutes. Be sure to hold each stretch for 15 to 30 seconds in order to gain maximum elongation in the muscle and minimize injury.

Cooling Down with the Ball

The exercises in this section

- ✔ Loosen your hip joints
- ✔ Stretch your muscles
- ✔ Elongate your spine
- ✔ Slow your heart rate
- ✔ Help your blood flow back to your muscles, heart, and lungs when you're done working out

I encourage you to breathe through each exercise, taking notice of how your heart rate drops as you enjoy the wonderful relaxation that comes over your body when you're done.

Make sure that you're in *neutral spine* (or using a flat back) when you do the reach-and-release and spinal rotation exercises in this section. Maintaining a neutral spine keeps you from placing strain on your lower back and ensures a good stretch.

Hip circles

Hip circles release built-up tension in your hip joint, which helps loosen up the pelvis. This exercise is also a good beginning ball exercise because it helps familiarize you with sitting on the ball.

To do this exercise, follow these steps:

1. **Sit tall on the ball with your feet shoulder-width apart (as Figure 10-1a shows).**

2. **With your arms at your sides, slowly circle your hips to the right, pressing the ball into the ground (see Figure 10-1b).**

3. **Repeat two or three circles to the right and then repeat the movement on your left side.**

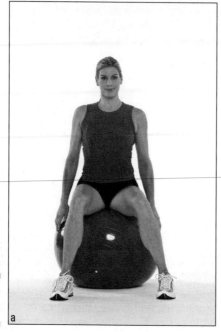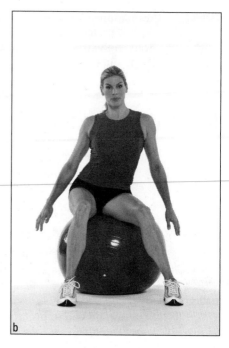

Figure 10-1:
Hip circles.

Complete five repetitions on each side.

Some do's and don'ts for this exercise:

✔ *Do* circle your hips slowly to loosen up your entire hip area.

✔ *Don't* let your feet leave the ground at any time during this exercise.

Back roll-up

The back roll-up loosens your upper back muscles, so take your time and roll up slowly.

To do this exercise, follow these steps:

1. **Sit on the ball with your hands on your thighs and look straight ahead (as Figure 10-2a shows).**

2. **Keeping your back straight, lean forward from your hips and hold the position for a moment.**

3. **Let your head and neck relax down toward your chest as you start rolling up your back and spine one vertebra at a time (see Figure 10-2b).**

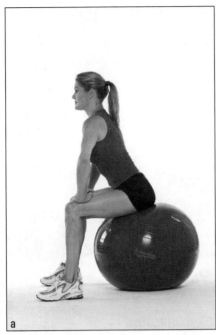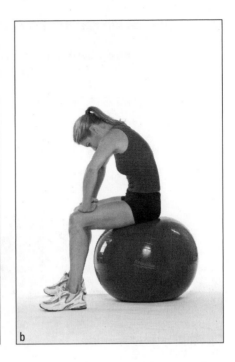

Figure 10-2:
Back
roll-up.

4. Finish the movement by lifting your head up slowly and rolling your shoulders back and down.

Complete two to three times.

A few do's and don'ts for this exercise:

✔ *Do* make sure you roll up slowly, one vertebra at a time.

✔ *Don't* tense up your shoulders. Keep them relaxed and pressed down during this exercise.

Shoulder stretch

The shoulder stretch stretches your chest muscles and the muscles in front of your shoulder. You can stretch one shoulder at a time or both shoulders at once. In the following steps, I tell you how to stretch both shoulders at the same time.

To do this exercise, follow these easy steps:

1. **Kneel behind the ball with your arms stretched out in front of you (as Figure 10-3 shows).**

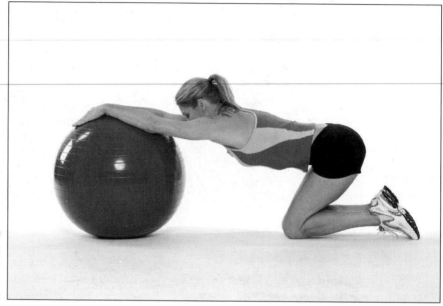

Figure 10-3:
Shoulder
stretch.

Place only one arm on the ball for an individual stretch and then alternate sides.

2. **Breathe out as you relax your body toward the floor, stretching your shoulder muscles.**

Hold this stretch for a few seconds before you release your body back up. Repeat this stretch two or three times.

A few do's and don'ts for this exercise:

- ✔ *Do* allow your head and neck to relax down toward the floor by casting your eyes downward.

- ✔ *Do* exhale with effort as you relax your body and stretch toward the floor.

- ✔ *Don't* let the ball move. Keep it steady and directly underneath your arms.

Backbend stretch

The backbend stretch is a good way to keep you from getting that stiff feeling in your back after a workout. It not only releases any tension from your back, but it also leaves you feeling revitalized.

Because your head is lower than your body during this exercise, take a few moments to rest between each back stretch so you don't feel dizzy from all the extra blood that's going to your brain!

To do this exercise, follow these steps:

1. **Lie face up and drape your body over the ball, keeping your knees bent and your feet flat on the floor (see Figure 10-4a).**

2. **Open your arms out to your sides in an airplane position and extend your legs in front of you, rolling the ball out slightly (as Figure 10-4b shows).**

3. **Drop your hips and bend your knees to come back to starting position.**

Complete ten repetitions.

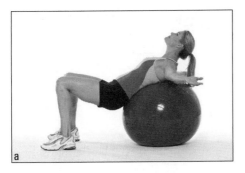

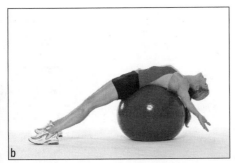

Figure 10-4:
Backbend
stretch.

A couple of do's and don'ts for this exercise:

- ✔ *Do* keep your eyes staring at the ceiling to keep your head from relaxing too far toward the ground.
- ✔ *Don't* let your feet come off the ground as you stretch your weight behind you.

Reach and release

This stretch is a good one because it leaves you feeling taller and gives you a total body stretch.

To get a better stretch, make sure you inhale and exhale a few times before you extend your arms over your head.

To do this exercise, follow these steps:

1. **Lie on the floor with your back in neutral spine and your legs out in front of you.**

   Point your toes to ensure that you get a good stretch from head to toe.

2. **Inhale as you place the ball overhead and stretch out your arms as far as you can with the ball behind you (as Figure 10-5 shows).**

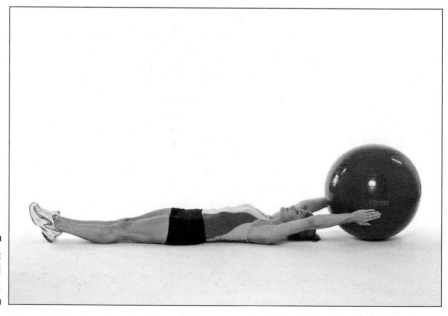

Figure 10-5:
Reach and
release.

3. **Exhale as you relax your arms farther behind your body.**

Complete this stretch five times.

A few do's and don'ts for this exercise:

- ✔ *Do* keep the ball resting on the floor behind you and not lifted off the ground.
- ✔ *Do* breathe deeply during this exercise.
- ✔ *Don't* forget to point your toes, which gives you an extra stretch along the entire length of your body.

Spinal rotation

A spinal rotation is a good way to end a workout because it stretches the muscles in your lower back along your spine. It also helps stimulate your immune system by releasing any extra energy you may have and distributing it throughout your body.

The key to this exercise is keeping your upper body flat and relaxed on the floor as you allow your knees to slowly roll from side to side.

To do this exercise, follow these easy steps:

1. **Lie flat on the floor with your knees bent and rest your hands on the ball above your head.**
2. **Slowly roll your knees to the right side as you roll the ball slightly to your left side (see Figure 10-6).**

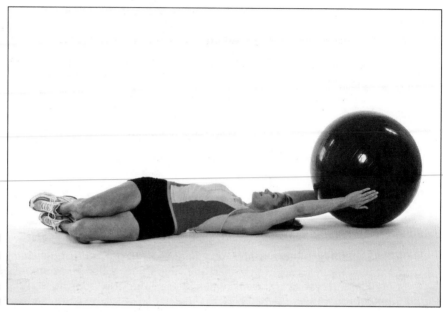

Figure 10-6:
Spinal
rotation.

3. **Exhale as you relax your back into the floor and feel the release of your hips and lower back.**

4. **Slowly roll your knees to the opposite side, remembering to keep your feet on the floor.**

5. **Hold the position for a few breaths before repeating on the other side.**

Complete a few repetitions on each side.

A few do's and don'ts for this exercise:

- ✔ *Do* take a few breaths slowly as you hold your stretch.

- ✔ *Do* keep your hands holding the ball on the floor above your head as you roll from side to side.

- ✔ *Don't* let your knees drop to the floor too fast. Instead, use a slow and controlled movement.

The drape

Many chiropractors love the drape exercise because it naturally stretches your back muscles by using your own weight placed over the ball. Adding a gentle rock to the drape is soothing and gentle.

To do this exercise, follow these steps:

1. **Kneel behind the ball and rest your arms at your sides.**

2. **Drape your body over the ball face down, resting your fingertips and your feet on the floor for support (as Figure 10-7 shows).**

   Let your head and neck relax to the floor.

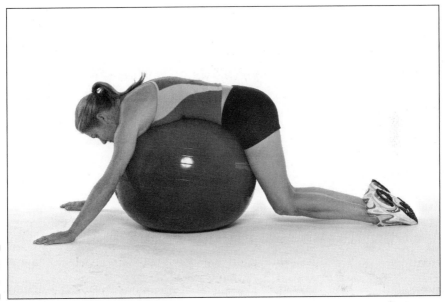

Figure 10-7:
The drape.

3. **Rock back and forth gently to release any built up tensions or tight muscles in your back.**

4. **Return to your starting position and rest on your knees before repeating the stretch.**

Repeat three to five times.

A couple of do's and don'ts for this exercise:

✔ *Do* let your body relax to the floor during this exercise.

✔ *Don't* forget to breathe, which allows your back muscles to release farther toward the floor.

✔ *Don't* forget to let your head and neck hang down in a relaxed position.

Stressed out?

One of the greatest sources of stress today is cramming your schedule and your children's schedules so full of activities that your head spins — figuratively and literally speaking. Exercise can cut your stress level in half and lower your blood pressure, which isn't a bad combination. Here are a few tips you can use to help you get back on track or just to encourage you to slow down a little:

✔ Do yoga, Pilates, or take the time to stretch to ease your body of aches and rid you of tension. Plus, it may even help you take a few much-needed breaths.

✔ Because stress is cumulative, reevaluating where you are in your life and making small changes along the way can really make a difference that shows up on a daily basis.

✔ Downsizing to a smaller company, taking on less of a work load, delegating chores to a relative or family member, or even moving to a smaller, tight-knit community may help you get back the simplicity you need in life to maintain a good, long, healthy life.

Chapter 11

Total Body Workout-in-One

. . . .

In This Chapter
▶ Getting the best placement for the ball and your body
▶ Warming up for a total body workout
▶ Ball exercises that work you from head to toe
▶ Cooling down from a total body workout

. . . .

This chapter is great for a total body workout, especially if you're short on time. When you can do this workout comfortably two or three days a week, you need to increase your resistance by adding weights or by using one of the accessories shown in Chapter 16.

If you want to work a particular area of the body or you want to focus on arms one day and legs the next, the specialized chapters in this book are better suited for you.

Adding cardiovascular training to go along with the total body workout is ideal. Alternating strength training and aerobic training is the best combination — sort of like a one-two punch to the body. However, nothing's wrong with doing both on the same day.

When you begin using exercise balls in your fitness program, you'll soon discover that they require a lot of endurance. Like with any new form of exercise, avoid overtraining by resting 24 to 48 hours in between workouts.

Positioning Yourself on the Ball

Training on the ball has its own unique challenges. Because of its round surface, the ball is able to mold to your body or roll away in some cases. Here are a few important points to keep in mind:

✔ Because some of the exercises in this chapter require balance and coordination, starting out with the ball placed against a hard surface for support can help you gain confidence while you become acquainted with

Working your core

You hear so much talk these days about working your "core," which people used to refer to as their midsection. The core is made up of the deep abdominal and back muscles that work as stabilizers for the entire body. These muscles are referred to as "deep" muscles because you can't see them. Still, these muscles are responsible for maintaining the body's core stability.

The three muscles in the core, or midsection or trunk, of the body are the *transverse abdominus, multifidus,* and the *quadratus lumborum.* These muscles work together to protect the spine and to help with everyday activities, such as lifting, throwing, bending, reaching, and running. So you

can see why keeping the stabilizer muscles well conditioned is extremely important.

Training on the ball is one way to reach this group of hard-to-find muscles. Just by sitting on the ball, you activate the stabilizer muscles and not only improve your posture, but you also gain a feeling of being more in touch with your center of gravity. Working your core is just one of the many benefits you get when you add exercise balls to your fitness program.

To work your core, try the exercises in Chapter 8, which are designed specifically for the chest, abs, and lower back.

the exercises in this chapter. Placing the ball against a wall or heavy couch may keep you from getting discouraged and give you a much better experience when you're just starting out on the ball.

✔ Just sitting on the ball is difficult because it's an unstable base that requires strength in your back and abdominal muscles. If you sit on a chair or a weight bench at the gym, you certainly don't use any of these muscles that you use when working out on the ball. By bringing your feet closer together when you're sitting on the ball, you can intensify your workout by altering your base of support.

✔ The farther away the ball is from your *core* (torso), the more difficult maintaining your balance is. For example, when you do a push-up on the ball, it's much easier when you place the ball underneath your lower legs because it's closer to your abs, hips, and glutes. To increase the difficulty, simply roll the ball out to your feet so that it's farther away from the center of your body, making maintaining your balance harder.

Warming Up for a Total Body Workout

For a quick warm-up that gets the heart pumping, I suggest a light five- to ten-minute workout of low-level cardio to increase body temperature and the flexibility of the muscles. Here are some suggestions for warming up the body:

✔ Jump rope for five minutes

Cross training

Cross training is essential in any exercise program because it keeps you from burning out or getting tired of one particular type of workout. If you're a runner who's used to running everyday, the muscles in your body will eventually reach a plateau, and you'll stop seeing improvement in your level of fitness.

Switching up your workout or trying something new is a good idea when you've been consistently training in one area. If you're a swimmer, try taking a step aerobics class. If you're a cyclist or are into spinning, try working the upper body by lifting weights or using resistance bands. A weight lifter can try taking a yoga or Pilates class to stretch out his muscles and add some flexibility to his workout. Avoiding boredom and keeping your fitness regimen new and fresh provides your body with changes that may surprise you.

✔ Get on a stationary bike for ten minutes

✔ Walk on a treadmill for ten minutes at a slow to moderate pace

✔ Walk outdoors, starting with a slow pace and working up to a faster pace

✔ Swim for half a mile

If you have a few extra minutes to spare and want a really great warm-up that uses the ball, head to Chapter 5.

Warming up your body increases the temperature of your muscles, which reduces the risk of injury.

Best-Bang-For-Your-Buck Workout

This workout provides crossover benefits for many of the activities you do in everyday life by mimicking the movements you use when you push, pull, kneel, or squat. In addition, these exercises help improve your overall strength.

The first six exercises in this section focus on working the upper body and training your core. The last six exercises in this section — including the wall squat, single-leg bridge, and leg curls — focus on working the lower body — your hips, thighs, and butt. For many people, especially women, this area is a big problem because of the large muscle groups involved here.

If you find the following exercises challenging but are able to maintain proper form while doing them, then you're working out at the right level for you.

When you're working with the ball, notice where your body is in relation to the ball. When you're just starting out, you may want to keep the ball as close to your core as possible to decrease the challenge and maintain your balance. As you become stronger and more confident with your ball workout, you can increase the difficulty by moving the ball further away from your body's core muscles.

Side reaches

Side reaches not only stretch the side muscles that run along the rib cage, but they also loosen up the entire body to prepare you for your workout.

To do this exercise, follow these steps:

1. **Sit tall and slightly forward on the ball. Rolling the ball to the right, extend your left leg, reaching over your head with your left arm (as Figure 11-1 shows).**

   Keep your right hand on your thigh and your left leg bent to support your weight on the ball.

2. **Straighten back to starting position and repeat on the other side.**

Complete five reaches for each side.

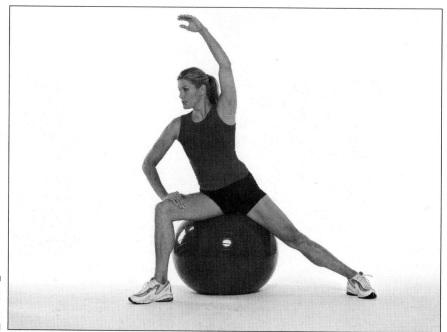

Figure 11-1:
Side reach.

A few do's and don'ts for this exercise:

✔ *Do* sit slightly forward on the ball. Doing so makes getting a complete stretch easier.

✔ *Don't* reach too far to the side because you may lose your balance.

Hip circles

Hip circles loosen up the pelvis by releasing any built-up tension in the hip joints. This exercise also helps you get used to sitting on the ball.

To do this exercise, follow these steps:

1. **Sit tall on the ball with your feet shoulder-width apart (see Figure 11-2a).**

2. **With your arms at your sides, slowly circle the hips to the right, pressing the ball into the ground (see Figure 11-2b).**

3. **Repeat two or three circles to the right, and then repeat the movement on your left side.**

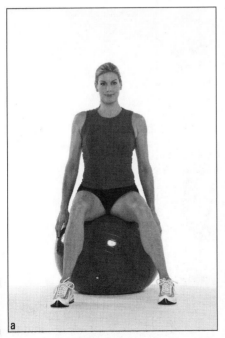
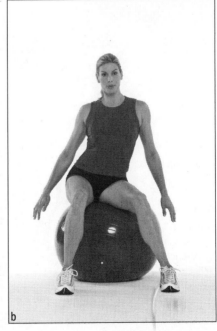

Figure 11-2:
Hip circles.

a

b

Some do's and don'ts for this exercise:

- ✔ *Do* circle the hips slowly to loosen up the entire hip area.
- ✔ *Don't* let your feet leave the ground at any time during this exercise because you may lose your balance and fall off.

Abdominal crunch

Doing abdominal crunches with the ball places the emphasis not only on the abs but also on the legs, butt and hips. By grasping the ball between your knees, the larger abdominal muscles or outer abdominals, get used a lot more intensely during this exercise.

To do this exercise, follow these steps:

1. **Lying on the floor, rest your lower legs on the ball at a 90-degree angle (see Figure 11-3a).**

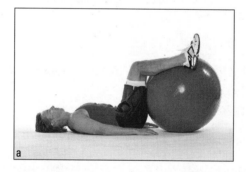

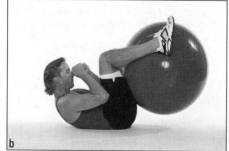

Figure 11-3:
Abdominal
crunch.

2. **As you tighten your abdominals, grasp the ball between your legs and pull toward you, lifting the ball from the floor.**

3. **With your hands on either side of your head, slowly lift your shoulders from the floor toward your knees (see Figure 11-3b).**

4. **Hold the lift for a few seconds and slowly roll your shoulders back to the floor.**

Complete ten repetitions.

A few do's and don'ts for this exercise:

✔ *Do* relax your neck as you curl up into a crunch.

✔ *Don't* forget to exhale as you curl up into the crunch and inhale as you release back down.

Ball lift with a twist

Because of the twisting motion in this exercise, your waist and oblique muscles get a workout along with your abs.

To do this exercise, follow these easy steps:

1. **Lie with your back on the ball and your feet planted firmly in front of you.**

   Make sure that you have your heels directly below your knees.

   Your shoulders don't touch the ball, so they're free to move from side to side.

2. **Place your arms criss-crossed on top of your chest (see Figure 11-4a).**

3. **Starting with your right shoulder, contract your abdominal muscles as you slowly lift and turn your body toward your left hip (see Figure 11-4b).**

4. **Stay lifted for a moment, and then slowly lower your body down to the starting position.**

5. **Slowly lift your left shoulder as you contract your abdominal muscles and turn your body toward your right hip.**

Continue alternating your right and left side lifts, doing two sets of 12.

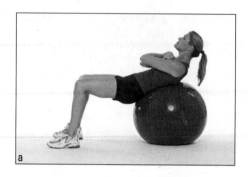

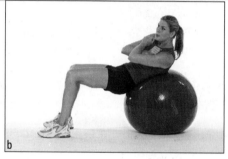

Figure 11-4:
Ball lift with
a twist.

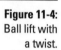

A few do's and don'ts to keep in mind:

- ✔ *Do* exhale before you contract your abdominal muscles and lift.

- ✔ *Do* inhale as you release your back down onto the ball in starting position.

- ✔ *Don't* rush through this exercise. Take a moment to pause at the top of the lift.

Alternating biceps curls

Biceps curls become much harder when you do them on the ball because of the instability factor. Concentrate on maintaining your balance throughout this exercise.

Beginners need 3- to 5-pound weights. Advanced men and women may use heavier dumbbells.

To do this exercise, follow these steps:

1. **Sit on the ball with your feet shoulder-width apart. Hold your weights down by your sides with your palms facing inward.**

2. **Pull in your abdominal muscles as you slowly bring your right weight toward your right shoulder (see Figure 11-5).**

   Your palm will be facing in toward your shoulder.

3. **Hold this movement for a few beats, and then release the weight back down to your right side. Repeat with your other arm.**

Complete two sets of ten repetitions.

A few do's and don'ts for this exercise:

✔ *Do* concentrate on your biceps muscles as you do this exercise.

✔ *Do* contract your abs before you lift the weight to your shoulder.

✔ *Don't* jerk the weight up to your shoulder. Use a slow and controlled movement.

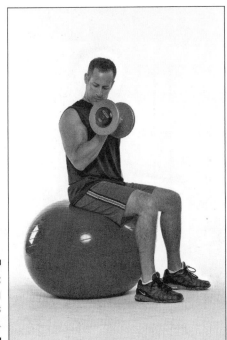

Figure 11-5:
Alternating
biceps
curls.

Triceps press

The triceps press works — you'll never believe this one — the *triceps,* or the back of the arms. When done on the ball, this exercise (which is usually done while sitting on a weight bench) becomes more challenging because you have to maintain your balance.

If you have a history of neck or shoulder problems, you may want to consult your doctor before trying this exercise, because lifting the weight behind your head can place strain on the back of your neck.

Beginners need a 3- to 5-pound weight. Advanced men and women may use a heavier dumbbell.

To do this exercise, follow these steps:

1. **Sit on the ball with your feet shoulder-width apart. Hold the weight in both hands behind your head (as Figure 11-6a shows).**

   Keep your elbows close to your forehead.

2. **Straighten your elbows, pressing the weight toward the ceiling (see Figure 11-6b).**

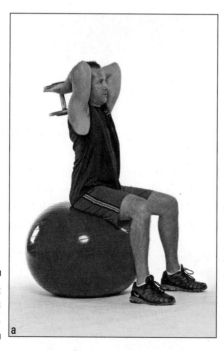
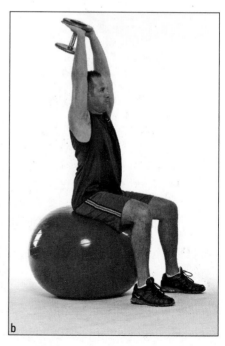

Figure 11-6:
Triceps
press.

3. **Bend your elbows to slowly lower the weight back down behind your neck.**

Complete two sets of ten repetitions.

A few do's and don'ts for this exercise:

✔ *Do* hold the weight in both hands behind your head.

✔ *Do* extend your elbows fully when you're pressing the weight above your head.

✔ *Don't* move your feet at any time. Keep them firmly planted on the ground.

✔ *Don't* forget to contract your abs before lifting the weight above your head.

When you do this exercise, think about pressing the weight upward, not forward or in front of your body. Doing so helps place the emphasis on the triceps. As you press the weight toward the ceiling, keep your elbows close to your forehead.

Torso lift

The torso lift helps improve posture and strengthens all the muscles along the spine. Doing the torso lift after working on your abdominal muscles also feels really good because of the opposing motion — lifting up rather than curling in.

To do this exercise, follow these steps:

1. **Lie with your stomach and waist on the ball and your legs extended behind you (see Figure 11-7a).**

   Make sure that you're resting the balls of your feet on the floor.

2. **As you exhale, extend your arms out to the side and lift your upper body toward the ceiling, straightening your back (see Figure 11-7b).**

3. **Hold this position for a few beats and then lower as you inhale.**

Complete ten repetitions, pausing for a few beats in between lifts.

A few do's and don'ts for this exercise:

✔ *Do* remember to exhale as you lift up to the ceiling.

✔ *Do* keep the balls of your feet on the floor.

✔ *Don't* arch your back. You want to keep your spine straight and long.

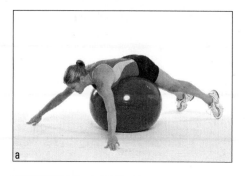

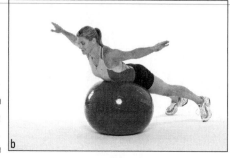

Figure 11-7:
Torso lift.

Backbend stretch

The backbend stretch feels really good right after you do abdominal crunches because by bending backward on the ball, you stretch your muscles in the opposite direction, reversing the motion of the crunch. This exercise also releases any tensions in your back that may have built up.

To do this exercise, follow these steps:

1. **Lying face up, drape your body over the ball with your knees bent and your feet flat on the floor (see Figure 11-8a).**

2. **Open your arms out to your sides in an airplane position and extend your legs in front of you, rolling the ball out slightly (as Figure 11-8b shows).**

3. **Drop your hips and bend your knees to come back down into starting position.**

Complete ten repetitions.

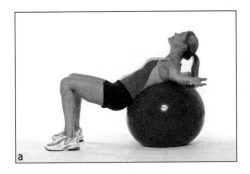

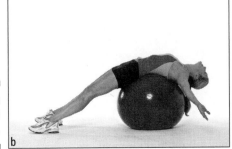

Figure 11-8: Backbend stretch.

A couple of do's and don'ts for this exercise:

✔ *Do* keep your eyes staring straight up at the ceiling to keep your head from relaxing down too far toward the ground.

✔ *Don't* forget to rest in between each repetition so you don't get dizzy from your head being lower than your body.

The bridge

The bridge is one of the most classic positions for ball exercises. It works the hips and lower back as you lift up your body.

To do this exercise, follow these steps:

1. **Rest your head and shoulders on the ball with your knees bent at a 90-degree angle (see Figure 11-9a).**

   Make sure that your knees are stacked over your ankles.

2. **Keep your arms folded behind your head and press the hips up toward the ceiling as high as possible (see Figure 11-9b).**

3. **Slowly lower your hips down to starting position.**

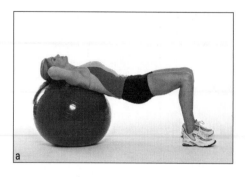

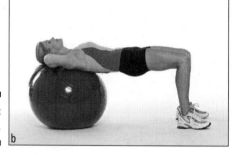

Figure 11-9:
The bridge.

Complete this exercise ten times.

A few do's and don'ts for this exercise:

✔ *Do* rest the back of your head on the ball during this exercise.

✔ *Don't* let your thighs and butt sink toward the ground. Keep everything tight and pressed upward during this exercise.

Wall squats

By placing the ball between you and a wall, a standard squat position becomes a wall squat. This exercise is great for working the *quadriceps* (front of the legs) and the butt.

To do this exercise, follow these steps:

1. **Place the ball between the wall and your lower back, walking your feet out slightly.**

2. **Lower your body toward the floor in a squat position as you continuously push back into the ball (see Figure 11-10).**

   Bend your knees to 90 degrees or as far as feels comfortable to you.

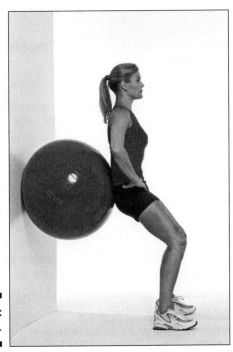

Figure 11-10:
Wall squat.

3. **Straighten your legs, keeping your weight over your heels to return to standing position.**

Complete 10 to 15 repetitions.

A couple of do's and don'ts for this exercise:

✔ *Do* keep your feet pointing straight forward as you lower into a squatting position.

✔ *Don't* let your knees roll out to the sides. Keep them in line with the rest of your body.

Push-ups

Push-ups on the ball target your chest muscles along with the abdominal muscles and butt to keep you steady on the ball.

Keeping your lower legs or shins on the ball will help you balance yourself during the push-up.

To do this exercise, follow these steps:

1. **Lie with your belly on the ball and walk your hands forward until the ball rests under your legs (as Figure 11-11a shows).**

   Make sure that your hands are directly below your shoulders on the floor.

2. **Lower toward the floor with the upper body, bending your elbows out to the side (see Figure 11-11b).**

3. **Straighten your elbows and exhale as you press back up into starting position.**

Complete ten repetitions.

A couple of do's and don'ts for this exercise:

✔ *Do* keep your abdominal muscles tight to help you maintain your balance.

✔ *Do* use proper breathing, inhaling as you lower and exhaling as you press back up.

✔ *Don't* arch your back. Keep it straight and in line with your head and the rest of your body.

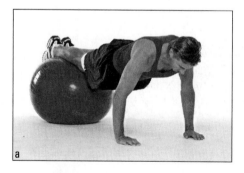

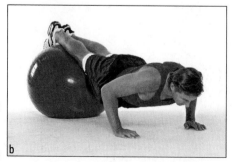

Figure 11-11:
Push-ups.

Single-leg bridge

A variation on the classic bridge, the single-leg bridge targets the hamstrings and glutes. Because the single-leg bridge uses the weight of only one leg to support the weight of your entire body, the all-important core muscles (abs and butt muscles) also get a good workout.

To do this exercise, follow these steps:

1. **Sit tall on the ball and roll down slowly until only your shoulders touch the ball (as Figure 11-12a shows).**

2. **As you contract your abs, place your left leg across your right thigh. Lift your hips up toward the ceiling as you contract your butt muscles (see Figure 11-12b).**

   If you find the ball moving at all during this exercise, place it against the wall or a heavy piece of furniture.

3. **Pause for a moment, and then lower your hips.**

Complete ten repetitions before switching legs and repeating on the other side.

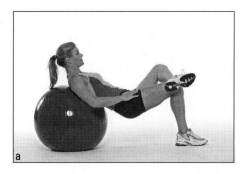

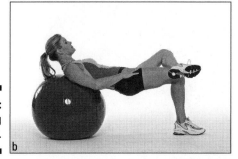

Figure 11-12:
Single-leg
bridge.

A couple of do's and don'ts for this exercise:

- ✔ *Do* keep your hands on your hips when doing this exercise to help steady your body.
- ✔ *Don't* press your hips too high. Keep them even with your torso.

Hamstring lift

Hamstring lifts work the entire lower body, which includes the hips, lower back, and legs. Because you use your feet and lower legs to control the movement of the ball, this exercise can also be a challenging one for your calf muscles.

To do this exercise, follow these steps:

1. **Lie on the floor with your feet placed on top of the ball (see Figure 11-13a).**

   Place your arms on the floor alongside your body for support.

2. **Exhale as you raise your hips and pelvis toward the ceiling, pressing down into the ball with your feet to maintain your balance (see Figure 11-13b).**

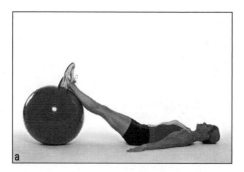

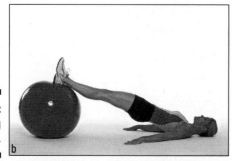

Figure 11-13: Hamstring lift.

3. Inhale as you slowly lower your hips back toward the floor.

Complete ten repetitions.

A few do's and don'ts for this exercise:

✔ *Do* keep your feet relaxed when they're resting on the ball.

✔ *Do* keep your back straight as you lift your hips.

✔ *Don't* lift your chin. Keep it tucked into your chest.

Leg circles

The lifting motion used by the hips in this exercise helps create a shapelier butt by defying gravity. By working the muscles in the upper leg and alongside the hips, you'll notice better buns in no time!

To do this exercise, follow these steps:

1. Lie on the floor, placing your left leg on the ball and extending your right leg toward the ceiling (as Figure 11-14a shows).

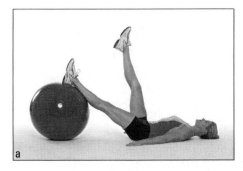

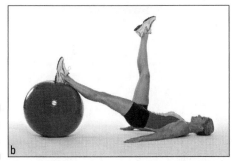

Figure 11-14:
Leg circles.

2. **Keeping your shoulders on the floor, lift your hips up, extending the leg straight above you. Pointing your toe, make five small circles to the right and then five small circles to the left (see Figure 11-14b).**

3. **Lower your leg down to the ball and return your hips to the floor. Repeat this movement on your other leg.**

Complete five sets on each leg.

A few do's and don'ts for this exercise:

✔ *Do* keep your arms flat on the floor alongside your body for support.

✔ *Don't* forget to contract your abs before lifting your hips off the floor.

✔ *Don't* tense your neck and shoulders as you lift the leg off the ball.

Finding neutral spine

So often you hear the term "neutral spine" used in exercise, but what is it? When your car is in neutral, you know that means it's in a "pause" mode, but does "neutral" mean the same thing in physiology?

Definitely not. Being in "neutral" is really an active position where the lower abdominal and pelvic stabilizer muscles are activated to create a "girdle" of sorts for the body to be able to protect itself from injury.

To keep your back from arching and to practice neutral spine, try this exercise in front of a mirror:

1. **Stand facing the side as you look into a mirror.**

2. **Now imagine a ruler extending down along your back from the top of your shoulders or shoulder blades to the bottom of your pelvis or hips.**

   You should be standing tall and straight with everything stacked up neatly as follows: head, shoulders, rib cage, pelvis, and legs.

You can also try this exercise by lying on the floor:

1. **Lie on the floor with your back pressed down.**

   If your back is flat, you shouldn't be able to put your hand between the floor and your back.

2. **Exhale as you bring your knees to your chest and think about the placement of your back on the floor.**

3. **Hold your knees to your chest for a few moments, and then release your legs back to the floor.**

   Notice how your back feels now. Is it pressed down, not arching? Can you feel the neutral position of your body as it relaxes on the floor but is actively pressed downward?

   You should now be able to slip your hand under your lower back and feel the natural curve of your spine, otherwise known as maintaining neutral spine.

You need neutral spine and the proper alignment with all exercise ball programs.

Cooling Down

Cooling down your body is equally as important as warming it up — maybe even more so. If you've ever stopped too quickly during an aerobic class or in the middle of a run, you know what I'm talking about. During a workout, the blood gets distributed to the extremities and needs time to return to the heart for oxygen. If you stop midstream, you can faint or get dizzy.

The best activity for cooling down your body after a workout is a five-minute, well-paced walk that ends in a slow-paced walk. Combine this with the easy cool-down moves in Chapter 10, and you're sure to feel relaxed and rejuvenated.

When you cool your body down properly, you minimize or eliminate the muscle soreness that can result from skimping on this important step.

Part III

Variety Is the Spice of Life: Doing Different Activities on the Ball

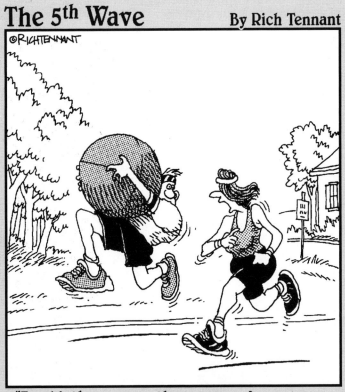

The 5th Wave   By Rich Tennant

"I said, there are other ways of getting an aerobic workout using an exercise ball."

In this part . . .

*T*he ball complements many different types of workouts. In Part III, I show you different ball exercises
that you can use with Pilates, yoga, stretching, and
choreographed cardio routines to burn extra calories.

Another option is to incorporate pieces of equipment —
such as medicine balls and resistance bands — into your
ball routine. This equipment increases your level of fitness by challenging your body through the use of new
exercise techniques. So, if accessorizing is your thing,
read Chapter 16 to find out how to use medicine balls and
resistance bands so you get more bang for your buck!

Chapter 12

Core Values: Pilates on the Ball

*P*ilates this, Pilates that — everywhere you go you can certainly find a Pilates class. Yes, the Pilates craze is upon us, and now that fitness gurus are combining it with the exercise ball, you can get a better, even more focused workout than before!

Adapting the Pilates method to the exercise ball makes sense for a variety of reasons. Here are some of the most important ones:

✔ Both Pilates and the exercise ball encourage working the core, or the entire torso, of the body.

✔ Both Pilates and the exercise ball are based in physiology for reforming injuries.

✔ Both Pilates and the exercise ball encourage using the deep stabilizing muscles of your body to achieve balance.

Pilates on the ball is a great example of one of the best fitness combinations you can do for your body.

This chapter takes some classic ball exercises and adds a Pilates twist, making them more intense — or should I say, more well-rounded?

Pilates Principles

The Pilates method has some basic principles, just as yoga (see Chapter 17) has some basic principles. The important point to remember here is that Pilates is a *mind and body* experience. It's not just a way to get in shape or reform injuries; it also creates a real awareness of how your body works and where all your movements originate.

The mindset you have when practicing Pilates is similar to the mindset of someone who's practicing martial arts. First, you must grasp the pebble from my hand, grasshopper. (I always loved that part in the television show, *Kung Fu*. And how true it is!) What I mean is that, in martial arts, you must first have the knowledge of the how and why to defend yourself before you go out and apply it. In Pilates, you must first understand the principles, or what you're trying to accomplish, before you do the exercise.

Here are the eight principles written by Joseph Pilates, the creator of Pilates, to help you perform his exercises as they were intended:

- ✔ **Breathing:** The best way to remember this principle is to exhale with effort. Using deep, diaphragmatic breathing (or breathing into your rib cage) allows you to create the proper flow and precision of each movement.

- ✔ **Range of motion:** This principle is basically flexibility, or how tight or loose your muscles are. Your range of motion affects your ability to stretch and extend, which are important to the Pilates method. People who have a limited range of motion will grow and benefit greatly from practicing Pilates.

- ✔ **Centering:** For this principle, you pull in your stomach muscles and engage your abdominals, working from your center for every movement. Centering is the basis for all Pilates work and for using the ball because it's an unstable base. Pulling your navel in toward your spine means sucking it in.

- ✔ **Controlling:** In this principle, you control your body's movements — each and every one of them. You know where everything is at all times. Having control of your body's movements creates body awareness that can enhance everything you do in life, from carrying a baby to stepping up on a ladder.

- ✔ **Stability:** For this principle, you want to *stabilize* your movements, or keep one body part still while another one is working. Stabilizing your lower back and not lifting your hips while you're lifting your legs is a good example of stability.

✔ **Flowing:** For this principle, you move freely through the movements, going from one to the next. The Pilates method has a real "dance" feel to it; you move smoothly through each exercise and finish with control.

✔ **Precision:** For this principle, you want to know where all your movements are coming from at all times. Being precise in each movement and being able to place your body and each limb where you would like it to be and where you would like it to end. Everything counts in Pilates and, for that reason, it takes a lot of focus and control to master it.

✔ **Opposition:** This principle is best described as working parts of your body in opposition to each other. Pressing your shoulders down while raising your arms or opening up your chest while bending at your waist are good examples of working in opposition.

To put all these principles together goes something like this: Teach your body to *flow* through movements with *precision* and *control*, working your body parts in *opposition* as you *breathe* through your limited *range of motion* and *centering* yourself as you *stabilize*.

The birth and explosion of the Pilates method

In the world of fitness, Pilates has exploded. Being a dancer, I was certified 12 years ago as a Pilates instructor. Most people who practice Pilates today think of it as something new when, in reality, it has been around for a long time.

Joseph Pilates, creator of the Pilates method, was born in 1881 and died in 1967. He was an accomplished circus performer, gymnast, and a notable boxer. Having many injuries from all the activities that he had participated in, Joseph Pilates came up with a series of exercises to overcome them. After perfecting these exercises that worked for him in rehabilitating his injuries, he wanted to pass this series of exercises onto ailing patients so they could recover, too, so he made crude pieces of equipment out of springs and pulleys to use with hospital beds. The result was that patients could get physical rehabilitation and work out while lying in bed. Genius!

Fast-forward many years later when Joseph Pilates turned these crude machines into what's now known as the Pilates *reformer,* or the Pilates *bed,* which can be used with more than 100 exercises devised by Joseph Pilates known as the *Pilates method*. The fact that the Pilates method today actually grew out of its roots and remained true to what it was created for is amazing. And, boy, is it ever still around today!

The art of Pilates has spread to athletes of all kinds along with professional dancers, and just about everybody in between. In fact, anyone who wants to create long, lean muscles and correct postural alignment problems is doing themselves a great service practicing Pilates. You can perform these exercises on an exercise mat (hence, the term *mat classes*), and you can use the mat exercises on the reformer.

To truly discover the who, what, where, when, and why of proper placement or where all these small movements come from, I recommend learning Pilates mat exercises first before adding any equipment.

Benefits of Combining Pilates with the Ball

You get some amazing benefits when you combine the ball and the Pilates method. Here are some of the most important benefits:

- ✔ Because the ball is difficult to keep still, it makes a great tool for teaching challenging exercises that require small movements and strength — like the Pilates method. In addition, the unstable base of the ball complements many of the Pilates-based exercises.

- ✔ Because the exercise ball is light and portable, it's easier to transport and more versatile compared with other pieces of Pilates equipment.

- ✔ You develop good muscle tone for your entire body. Because you're balancing the ball and recruiting major muscle groups, you train one muscle group while you use the other for balancing, which provides overall toning.

- ✔ You improve your flexibility. Ball stretches greatly improve the flexibility of your back and loosen tight hamstrings.

- ✔ You gain better posture and improve your balance by holding yourself steady on the ball and maintaining your balance.

- ✔ You strengthen your body's core. Using the ball trains your deeper abdominal muscles, which other pieces of fitness equipment don't.

- ✔ You can adapt it to your own level of fitness. You can easily modify ball exercises by keeping the ball closer to your torso or the core of your body. As you progress, move the ball away from your body's core toward your lower legs and feet to increase the difficulty.

- ✔ You improve your cardiovascular system and burn fat by using a low-impact workout. Ball exercises use so many muscles that they allow your heart rate to remain elevated throughout your workout.

Trade your chair for a ball?

In 1963, Italian toymaker Aquilino Cosani created the exercise ball, or "Swiss ball" as it was called then, as a colorful air-filled toy for children to play with. In the early 1980s, the exercise ball was sold to physical therapists and hospitals for purposes of patient rehabilitation. Today, exercise balls are still widely used throughout Europe for physical rehabilitation and physical fitness. In addition, many businesses and schools are seriously considering turning their chairs in for the ball. In fact, studies have shown that simply sitting on the ball enhances children's and employees' performances as well as concentration, posture, and organization.

Combining the principles and benefits of these two powerhouse forms of exercises can greatly improve your body's health. As with anything that's paired as a team, the results can be twice as good and twice as rewarding!

Before You Begin: Preparing for Pilates on the Ball

You need a few things before you can do the Pilates exercises in this chapter. In this section, you find a list of the items you need and what you can do to make your workout go more smoothly.

In this section, you also discover how to find the *neutral spine* position that you need to use for every exercise on the ball. Make sure you take the time to try this position before you begin your workout. Good luck!

Stuff you need

Here's the additional equipment you need to do Pilates on the ball:

✔ **Exercise mat:** You need an exercise mat to do the Pilates exercises in this chapter. An exercise mat allows you to kneel or lie on the floor so you can do the exercises more comfortably. It also prevents the ball, your feet, and your hands from slipping and sliding as you perform the exercises. A yoga mat works well or you can try a small slip-resistant rug.

✔ **Comfortable clothing that's somewhat fitted:** You don't want your clothing to be too loose because it can get caught in the ball. The same goes for long hair, so be sure to pull it back before you begin your workout.

Wearing something that allows you to see your stomach or abdominal muscles while working out is also a good idea so you can see whether you're breathing properly and keeping your rib cage open.

Stuff you don't need

Leave your shoes and socks off for these exercises, but save them for when you're using weights or doing cardio exercises on the ball. Because you need to grip the floor with your feet, going barefoot for this workout is best.

However, if you do feel yourself losing your balance and slipping around, try some light rubber-soled shoes to assist you until you become a bit more proficient on the ball.

Safety concerns

REMEMBER

To work out safely when you combine Pilates and the ball, keep the following points in mind:

✔ Make sure that you work out in a space that has few other objects in it so you can roll around comfortably and lie flat on the floor.

✔ Because you'll be using an exercise mat, don't forget to add in any additional space that you'll need. Using a non-slip surface is important so you can grip the floor with your fingers and toes and not lose control of the ball.

✔ Staying hydrated is vital to your workout. It helps you recharge and keeps you from building up lactic acid in your muscles. *Lactic acid* is what makes you sore at the end of an intense workout. Keep a water bottle handy so you can sip it throughout your exercise session — it'll provide you with better stamina so you can last longer on the ball.

✔ As with any new workout, consulting your physician before you begin a new workout is important. If at any time during this workout you feel any pain, stop what you're doing and rest quietly on your mat or stretch yourself over the ball for support. A good rule when exercising is, "if in doubt, leave it out!"

Finding that elusive neutral spine

One of the principle factors in practicing Pilates is *neutral spine.* The ultimate goal in trying to achieve a neutral spine is to keep the natural curve of your spine without overcorrecting it.

In other words, you want to stabilize your back, your hipbones, and your pelvis so they're on the same plane.

To try neutral spine and to see whether you're maintaining that natural curve in your spine, do the following:

1. **Lie with your back and feet flat on the floor and your knees bent at a 90-degree angle.**

2. **Flatten your lower back by pressing it into the floor.**

   Now you can feel the difference between neutral spine and a flat back.

3. **Arch your back slightly by lifting your hips up.**

   Now you can feel the differences between an arched back, a flat back, and the natural curve in your spine (or neutral spine).

If you were standing, your pelvis would drop straight down. The proper way to describe a neutral spine while standing up would be neither arched nor tilted forward. Just as your car has a neutral position in which it doesn't move forward or backward, the same goes for a neutral spine.

Getting Down to Business: Pilates on the Ball Exercises

This series of exercises starts with a breathing technique to help you create the body awareness you need to get you through this workout. And don't forget: *Breathing* is one of the eight Pilates principles. The plank and the bridge are modified ball exercises that require *stamina* and *balance*. And even a few more of your Pilates principles, such as *centering* and *opposition,* appear here. The last two exercises — the roll down and the back stretch — require great focus and *stability* because you need to keep the ball still as you lay across it, over it, and roll down it.

You should perform these exercises in the following order to allow your chest to open up before you release your back.

Diaphragmatic breathing with the ball

By placing the ball on your belly, the exercise ball can help you become more aware of the area you're using to breathe. As you inhale, you can see the ball rise as your belly fills with air and as you exhale, you can see the ball fall.

Rather than using your hand to feel your abdomen and rib cage rise, try using the ball.

To do this exercise, follow these steps:

1. **Lie on your back and bend your knees, keeping your feet flat on the floor.**

   Your legs should be hip-distance apart.

2. **Rest the ball on your belly and against your knees. Support the ball with your hands on either side (as Figure 12-1 shows).**

3. **Take a deep breath, allowing the ball to rise as your belly fills with air.**

4. **Exhale, making sure that all the air leaves your belly.**

5. **Repeat immediately after your exhale.**

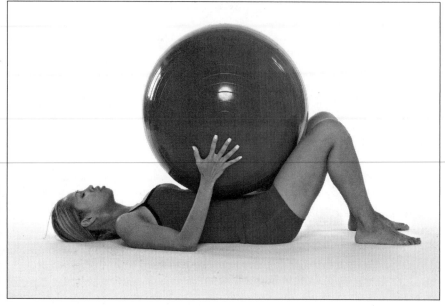

Figure 12-1:
Diaphrag-
matic
breathing
with
the ball.

Inhale to the count of ten and exhale to the count of ten for several breaths.

A few do's and don'ts for this exercise:

✔ *Do* keep your back pressed into the floor so you can feel your rib cage expand.

✔ *Do* inhale through your *nose.*

✔ *Don't* forget to keep your legs hip-distance apart to make room for the ball to move freely when you breathe.

The plank

The *plank* position and exercise is just how it sounds: You keep your body straight in a plank position, or rigid like a plank of wood. (I find that using analogies can help you remember poses or positions.)

Plank on the ball works your core muscles while it also works your upper body. It strengthens and lengthens your body by activating your stabilizing muscles as you slightly roll back and forth on the ball.

To do this exercise, follow these steps:

1. **Roll out onto the ball so your tummy is positioned in the center of it.**

2. **With your hands pressed down and your fingers facing forward, place your hands shoulder-width apart on the floor in front of you (as Figure 12-2 shows).**

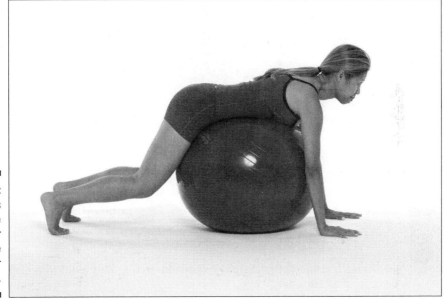

Figure 12-2:
Your hands
should be
on the floor
and in line
with your
shoulders.

Your arms will be straight underneath your shoulders.

3. **Slowly lift your legs behind you and onto the ball, creating a straight line down the center of your body, or a plank position (see Figure 12-3).**

   You need to contract your chest muscles and engage your upper body for additional support.

4. **Squeezing your butt muscles and pulling your belly button in, slightly rock your body forward to the front of the ball.**

   Your knees will be on top of the ball, making maintaining the plank position harder.

5. **Hold this position for a few seconds before rocking your body back a few inches in the opposite direction.**

6. **Bring your hands and arms back into the ball and rest before repeating.**

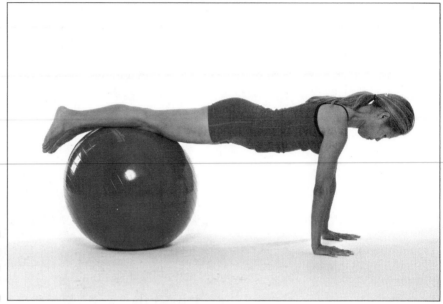

Figure 12-3:
Stay stiff as
a board!

Complete five to ten repetitions, depending on your individual fitness level.

Some do's and don'ts for this exercise:

- ✔ *Do* bring the ball closer to your torso if rolling it out to your knees is too difficult.
- ✔ *Do* press into the floor and squeeze your glutes while you're in the plank position.
- ✔ *Do* keep your neck in line with your spine as you do when you're standing.
- ✔ *Don't* let your back arch or sag. Keep it straight and long.

The bridge

The Pilates bridge on the ball is a variation of the classic bridge position that Chapter 9 illustrates. The version on the ball is more difficult because you have to control the ball and keep it steady using only your feet.

You need to incorporate your core muscles (remember, from your rib cage to your hips) or stabilizers to help you maintain control of the ball throughout this exercise.

To do this exercise, follow these steps:

1. **Place your lower legs and feet on the ball as you lie on the floor (see Figure 12-4).**

   Your arms will be straight and alongside your body.

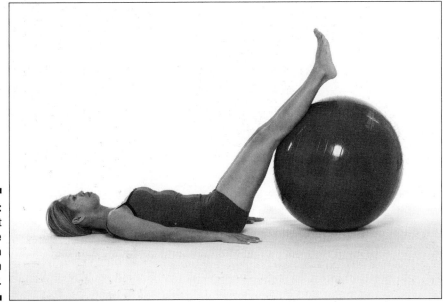

Figure 12-4:
Your feet
are on the
ball when
you lie on
the floor.

2. **As you inhale, contract your glutes as you lift up your hips and press your feet down into the ball (as Figure 12-5 shows).**

   Be sure not to place any strain on your neck by lifting too high. Lift up only as high as hip level.

3. **Hold for a few seconds using the support of your arms and your breathing to help you maintain the position.**

4. **Exhale as you slowly roll your spine back down onto the floor one vertebra at a time.**

Complete five to ten repetitions, depending on your individual fitness level.

A few do's and don'ts for this exercise:

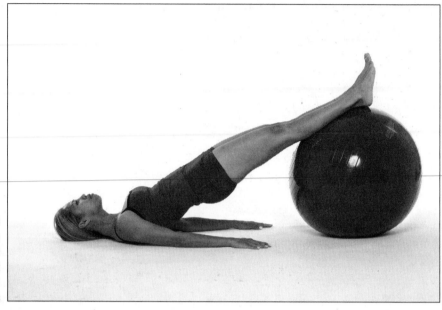

- ✔ *Do* inhale as you lift up your hips.
- ✔ *Do* keep your eyes cast toward the ceiling to help you keep your neck straight during the lift.
- ✔ *Don't* let the ball roll out from under you. Control it by pressing your feet down into it.

Roll downs

The roll down exercise is just as it sounds. Using a slow and controlled movement, you roll down onto the ball and then back up. This exercise helps you develop strong abdominal and lower back muscles, which help you maintain a strong and healthy back.

Using an exercise mat under the ball for the roll down exercise makes controlling the ball easier.

To do this exercise, follow these steps:

1. **Sit tall on the ball with your feet a little wider than hip-distance apart.**

2. **Pulling your belly button in toward your spine to activate your abdominal muscles, extend your arms straight out in front of you (as Figure 12-6 shows).**

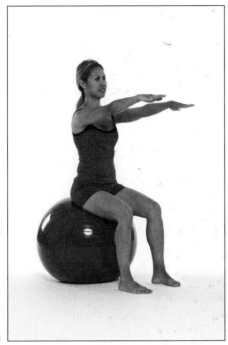

Figure 12-6:
Sitting tall
on the ball
with arms
out in front
of you.

3. **Slowly roll the ball forward using your tailbone until your shoulders and upper back are resting on the ball (see Figure 12-7).**

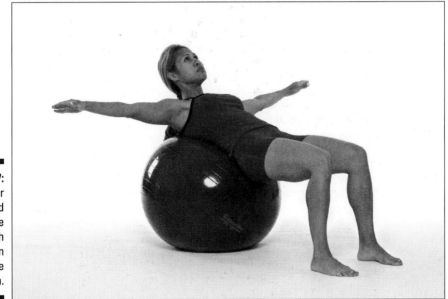

Figure 12-7:
Your upper
back should
be on the
ball with
your arms in
an airplane
position.

You will need to step your feet out in front of you to make room for the ball when it rolls forward.

4. **Inhale as you open your arms to the sides in an airplane position.**

5. **Exhale as you bring your arms back in front of your body at chest level.**

6. **Slowly roll yourself back up into starting position using the strength of your abs, glutes, and lower back.**

Your feet will be firmly planted on the ground as you stretch your arms forward.

Complete five repetitions.

A few do's and don'ts for this exercise:

✔ *Do* use a slow and controlled movement when rolling onto the ball.

✔ *Do* use your breath to help you focus on holding your position.

✔ *Don't* forget to use your exercise mat to get a better grip with your feet.

Back stretch

The backstretch opens up your chest and releases your back at the same time. This stretch is excellent for all levels.

The Pilates version of the back stretch is different than the classic back stretch in Chapter 10. Because you start from a squat-like position and lift back over the ball, this stretch requires extra support from your legs and uses the additional weight of your upper body as resistance.

To do this exercise, follow these steps:

1. **With your upper back on the ball, place your feet on the ground and your knees at a 90-degree angle.**

2. **Extend your arms behind your body to open up your chest (as Figure 12-8 shows).**

Your head and neck will rest on the ball for support.

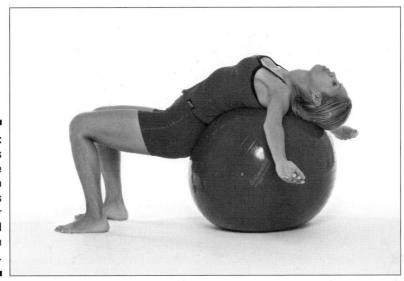

Figure 12-8:
Your thighs should be parallel to the floor as your upper back and head rest on the ball.

3. **Rolling the ball forward slowly, lower your butt toward the floor as you allow your knees to bend and open to a seated squat position (see Figure 12-9).**

   Your head and neck will still relax and lie on the ball for support.

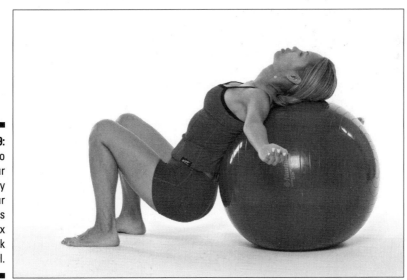

Figure 12-9:
Be sure to let your lower body support your weight as you relax your back on the ball.

Womb-like qualities of the ball

I can't believe how my baby just loves the ball! People always tell me that the ball seems familiar to her because it's like being back in the womb because of the shape or some other silly reason. And I'm sure being light and filled with air has something to do with it, too. However, when I saw my daughter (who's only 2 years old) run toward it with such excitement, I knew there had to be more to the story. And it turns out, there is!

According to the American College of Obstetricians, touch is a sense that develops inside the womb. Touching and playing with the ball gives us a memory of when this sense originally developed because the surface of the ball feels soft to the touch.

Draping your body over the ball, like in the drape exercises in Chapters 10 and 19, is one of the greatest sensations you can experience on the ball. Especially because achieving a perfect state of relaxation is so hard to do with all the noise and commotion that's going on in the outside world. The fact that a simple ball can bring us such joy and comfort is a wonderful thing.

For a deeper stretch, turn your feet and legs out to a *plie* position. (A plie is a ballet move that has become common with regular forms of exercise.) To perform a plie, turn your feet out to a 45-degree angle and descend toward the ground as you open your legs and knees out to the sides.

4. Hold your seated squat for 10 to 20 seconds as you inhale and exhale.

5. Use your heels to press back up to return to the starting position.

Complete five repetitions.

A few do's and don'ts for this exercise:

- ✔ *Do* keep your arms open to get a good stretch through the entire chest area.
- ✔ *Do* keep both feet flat on the floor to avoid slipping off the ball.
- ✔ *Do* keep your back pressed firmly into the ball for more control.
- ✔ *Don't* come up too fast after being in the seated squat position.

Chapter 13

Gaining Muscle Power: Weight Training

- -

In This Chapter

▶ Using weights in your ball program

▶ Ball exercises that enhance the benefits of weight training

▶ Getting the fluids your body needs during a workout

▶ Knowing the perfect amount of weight for you

- -

*T*his chapter contains a challenging and dynamic workout that uses heavier weights than you're probably used to training with. The workout consists of eight exercises that provide a total body workout by strengthening the abdominals, back, chest, and leg muscles.

In addition to requiring good balance and the use of your stabilizing muscles, these exercises use free weights to build overall body strength. When combined with the exercise ball, weights add a crucial element — the need to maintain good posture throughout each exercise. I use the exercise ball regularly to keep my back in good shape, but when I'm looking to build strong, lean muscles, I use the following workout that incorporates heavy dumbbells and ankle weights.

If you're looking for muscle endurance, you want to increase the repetitions and use lighter weights.

To avoid overtraining, never complete more than 20 weight-lifting sets during your workout. Also, be sure to rest three to five minutes between sets.

Bigger Muscles Burn More Fat!

With so much emphasis on cardio and dieting these days, building bigger muscles to lose weight is just starting to get the attention that it deserves. If you want to see your belly shrink, you need to make your muscles bigger and stronger. A weight-training workout burns more calories for the following reasons:

✔ Building bigger muscles boosts your *metabolic rate* (the rate at which your body burns calories).

✔ You burn 30 to 50 calories per day for each extra pound of muscle that you put on.

✔ Lean body mass burns more calories than fat body mass does.

To build bigger muscles, you need to work the larger muscle groups throughout your body. *Compound exercises,* which target more than one muscle group, such as squats, lat pulls, and chest presses, rather than exercises that target individual muscles, are great examples of ways to burn the most calories in the shortest amount of time.

R.I.C.E.

Rest, ice, compression, elevation — you've probably heard or read about using this prescription when you overdo it at the gym. But just when should you use ice and when should you use heat for overtired, overstrained muscles? Well, the truth is, both are great remedies for aches and pains. Ice reduces swelling, and heat increases the blood flow to your injured muscles, which speeds up circulation for faster healing.

Here are a few general rules to make your choice a little clearer:

✔ If the pain is minor, use ice for the first day or so; then use heat thereafter.

✔ If the pain is dull and achy, heat is best to work out the knots.

✔ If the pain is sharp, ice is best to reduce swelling.

✔ If you're really in pain, try alternating ice and heat for 20 minutes, but always end with ice.

Taking an over-the-counter anti-inflammatory drug like ibuprofen also works wonders to reduce inflammation. If the pain is moderate to severe, take every opportunity to get off your feet that you can. However, if your pain is minor, exercise can help the pain go away faster by strengthening the supportive muscles.

Swimming and walking are two excellent forms of exercise that you can do to get the blood flowing to the sore areas to expedite the healing process.

The Perfect Weights for You

Both men and women can benefit greatly from using weights. Most women are afraid they'll get too "big" if they lift weights. Honestly, it takes a lot of working out to do that. However, firming up various body parts is the biggest advantage to using the right amount of weight. But what's the right amount? Well, let me tell you.

The following weight amounts are recommended by the President's Council on Physical Fitness for use with the ball. At the gym, on a weight bench, or with machines, you want to increase the amount significantly.

Hand weights

For men and women who want to increase lean body mass and tone up, using enough weight that allows you to do 10 to 15 repetitions comfortably without causing exhaustion or strain is the right amount. For most women, this would be 10 to 15 pounds and for most men, this would be 25 pounds.

Ankle weights

Adding ankle weights to floor exercises increases the intensity and your fitness level. Besides increasing the gravitational pull while exercising, the extra weight works the glutes, hamstrings, calves, and quadriceps like never before. Most ankle weights start at 1½ pounds and go up to 15 pounds. The most popular and effective weight for women to use is somewhere between 2 and 10 pounds. For men, the most effective weight is from 10 to 15 pounds.

Dumbbells

For men and women interested in building muscle mass, heavier dumbbells that only allow you to do 6 to 8 repetitions is the perfect amount. For most people, around 25 pounds is the amount that you can use safely with the ball without sacrificing proper form.

Replenishing your fluids

If you do anything less than an hour of exercise, water will do just fine. If you're planning on exercising more than an hour, though, or if you sweat a lot, your body will need more than water. To be exact, something with a little bit of salt and a little bit of sugar to replace what you've lost.

Sports drinks are abundant in the market today, and they contain mainly sugar. A good do-it-yourself sports drink is an 8-ounce glass of water mixed with a tablespoon of sugar, a tablespoon of orange juice, and a pinch of salt. With all the choices out there to choose from, I personally don't know many people who take the time to make their own; however, it does help to know the ingredients of what you're drinking.

Energy drinks that contain ginseng, caffeine, and all kinds of other supplements for boosting energy levels have also become popular in the past few years. Some of these drinks have been known to have side effects, such as nausea or stomach cramps. I like sticking to things where I know what's in them rather than taking a chance on getting sick before a workout. But that's just my opinion.

Whatever you choose to drink before, during, or after a workout, remember that staying hydrated is important to your overall performance and health.

Here are the top-five signs of dehydration, in case you ever get to that point:

✔ Nausea after exercising

✔ Lightheadedness or dizziness after exercising

✔ Dark yellow urine or none at all

✔ Dry eyes (not tearing up)

✔ Dry, sticky mouth

Carrying a water bottle that you can replenish throughout the day is a good way to always ensure that you'll have a drink when you need one. Just don't reach for a soda — it's harder on the stomach and may give you that unpleasant bloated feeling from all the carbonation!

Bridge Poses

Challenging your core strength is the main goal of performing this group of exercises in conjunction with the bridge pose. While in a bridge position, all your core, or stabilizing, muscles get an intense workout from supporting your body weight as you lift it upward. In addition, the gravitational force of being in a lifted position creates strong hamstrings, quadriceps, and gluteal muscles.

The following exercises are intermediate exercises, and you should do them only when you feel that you're strong enough to perform them without letting your back sag or arch.

Warm up to power up

Begin any strength-training session with five to ten minutes of a light or low-level cardiovascular warm-up to increase core temperature throughout your entire body and to reduce the risk of injury. A cardiovascular warm-up also increases flexibility and elasticity in the muscles.

Another aspect of warming up your body before you begin weight training is practicing a light warm-up set. A light warm-up set consists of using half the amount of weight that you would normally use in your workout, which allows you to practice good technique and helps you avoid injury by getting your coordination together before you do any heavy lifting — especially when you're exercising on the ball. I can't emphasize enough how much extra effort you're going to have to make just to stay balanced while performing the following workout. Good luck!

Bridge with ankle weights

This exercise is all about lifting your legs against resistance. All your lower body muscles, including your glutes, hamstrings, calves, and quadriceps get a great workout.

Doing this exercise without shoes on is best because it makes keeping your feet positioned on the ball easier. You need 2- to 5-pound ankle weights for resistance.

Lie on an exercise mat to make your shoulders more comfortable when they're resting on the floor. Using a mat also helps keep the ball steady and prevents it from rolling away during this exercise.

To do this exercise, follow these steps:

1. **Wearing ankle weights, lie on the floor with your arms at your sides. Place your feet and lower legs comfortably on the ball.**

2. **Keeping the ball as still as possible, lift your pelvis toward the ceiling using your hamstring and gluteal muscles (see Figure 13-1).**

3. **Hold your body up and off the floor for a few seconds and then slowly return to the beginning position.**

   Be sure to inhale as you lift your body up and exhale as you lower it back to the floor.

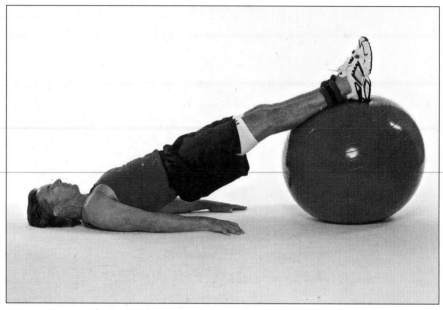

Figure 13-1:
Bridge
with ankle
weights.

Complete two sets of ten repetitions.

To strengthen your quadriceps and to increase the resistance of your workout, lift one leg off the ball and hold for a few seconds when your hips are lifted off the floor.

A couple of do's and don'ts for this exercise:

- ✔ *Do* keep the ball as still as possible by pressing down with your lower legs.
- ✔ *Don't* place strain on your neck muscles by hyperextending them. Keep your gaze up toward the ceiling and your neck in line with your spine.

Bridge with dumbbells and ankle weights

By adding a chest press to the bridge with ankle weights exercise, you ask the body to perform a multifunction. You have to maintain proper form on the ball while you work on maintaining your stability . . . much harder than it sounds, as you'll soon find out!

You can also do this exercise best without shoes on because it makes keeping your feet positioned on the ball easier.

For this exercise, you need 2- to 5-pound ankle weights for resistance. If you're an advanced exerciser, you need 10- to 15-pound hand weights.

To do this exercise, follow these steps:

1. **Wearing ankle weights and holding your dumbbells in your hands with your palms facing forward, lie with your back flat on the floor and your feet and lower legs resting on the ball.**

   You wear ankle weights to increase the resistance and to strengthen the muscle groups needed in this exercise.

2. **Slowly lift your pelvis up, keeping your elbows on the floor for support (as Figure 13-2a shows).**

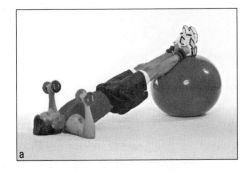

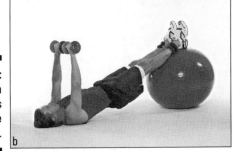

Figure 13-2:
Bridge with
dumbbells
and ankle
weights.

3. **Raise the dumbbells toward the ceiling, keeping them at chest level and your shoulders pressed down and into the floor (see Figure 13-2b).**

4. **Slowly lower your weights back to the starting position, keeping the ball still.**

Complete two sets of ten repetitions.

A few do's and don'ts for this exercise:

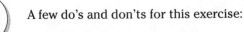

✔ *Do* keep your back straight and lifted during the chest press.

✔ *Do* keep the dumbbells at chest level.

✔ *Don't* forget to use your breath, inhaling as you lift up the pelvis and exhaling as you lower toward the floor.

Bridge with chest press

The chest press with a bridge combines two great exercises — the bridge and the chest press — to work the pectoral muscles along with the hips, butt, and hamstring muscles.

Be sure to keep your hips pressed toward the ceiling during this exercise. Any sagging or arching in your lower back can place unwanted strain on your back muscles.

To do this exercise, follow these steps:

1. **Rest your upper back on the ball with your knees bent at a 90-degree angle.**

   Make sure you keep your knees stacked over your ankles.

2. **With a weight in each hand, extend your arms toward the ceiling, placing the weights directly above your chest (see Figure 13-3).**

   Your palms will be facing forward as you press your weights up.

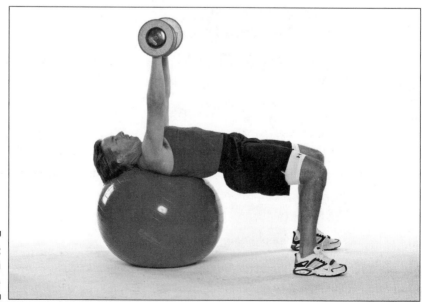

Figure 13-3:
Bridge with chest press.

3. Lower your weights by bending your elbows in toward your body.

Complete two sets of 10 to 15 repetitions.

A couple of do's and don'ts for this exercise:

✔ *Do* slowly press the weights up above your head, feeling your chest muscles contract.

✔ *Don't* let the ball move at all. Keep it steady.

Dumbbell Training Program

The next group of exercises works the upper body using weights with different ball positions to strengthen your muscles and improve your balance and alignment. By simply placing the ball between you and the wall, you will need to maintain your balance by tightening your abdominal muscles and keeping your back straight and long.

Standing biceps curls

This exercise adds a new twist to the simple biceps curl. I suggest starting off with 5-pound weights, because combining upper-body strengthening with lower-body toning can prove too challenging with heavy weights right off the bat. This exercise is a great way to target both areas at the same time.

Because keeping your feet steady may be difficult, be sure not to lose your balance by pressing your upper back into the ball.

To up the challenge, you can increase the weight and repetitions as you feel more comfortable.

To do this exercise, follow these steps:

1. Position the ball between your back and the wall. Pick up your dumbbells and hold them in your hands with your palms facing inward.

2. Lower your body slowly into a squat position (as Figure 13-4a shows).

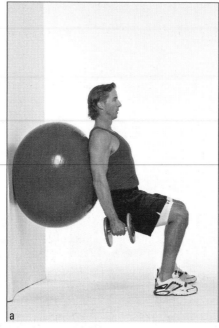
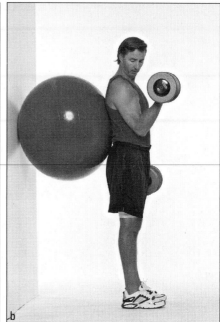

Figure 13-4:
Standing
biceps
curls.

a

b

3. **Slowly straighten back to the starting position as you curl your right bicep (refer to Figure 13-4b).**

4. **Repeat, this time curling your left bicep.**

Complete two sets of 10 to 15 repetitions.

A few do's and don'ts for this exercise:

- ✔ *Do* keep your back pressed into the ball as you straighten up into a standing position.

- ✔ *Do* straighten your arms fully after each biceps curl to get the full benefit of this exercise.

- ✔ *Don't* lean sideways at all during this exercise. Stand tall and straight, keeping the ball steady.

Standing rows

This exercise works your entire arm and shoulder. As you perform this exercise, maintaining proper form as you balance your knee on the ball is important.

To do this exercise, follow these steps:

1. **Place your right knee on the ball, keeping your upper torso almost parallel to the floor.**

2. **Balance yourself on the ball using your left hand and hold your weight in your right hand at your side (as Figure 13-5a shows).**

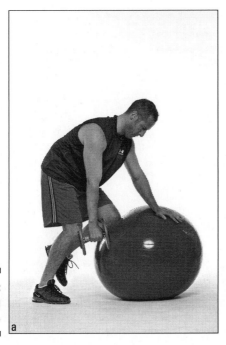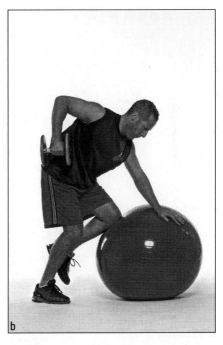

Figure 13-5:
Standing
rows.

a b

3. **Pull your weight up with a rowing motion as your elbow pulls back past your rib cage (as Figure 13-5b shows).**

4. **Hold for a few seconds and then release your weight back to your side.**

Complete ten repetitions and then switch sides and repeat.

A few do's and don'ts for this exercise:

✔ *Do* pull your elbow back as far as you can.

✔ *Don't* lift your head up because it causes your back to arch. Keep a long, straight spine during this exercise.

✔ *Don't* lose your balance. If this exercise proves too challenging, practice it off the ball first.

Squatting with dumbbells

This exercise strengthens your muscles by increasing the workload on your *quadriceps* (upper leg muscles). To meet the increased challenge of keeping the ball steady behind your back, you need to maintain neutral spine or keep your knees and toes in proper alignment.

To do this exercise, follow these steps:

1. **With your feet shoulder-width apart, stand with the ball between you and the wall behind your lower back. Hold your dumbbells down by your sides (as Figure 13-6a shows).**

Figure 13-6:
Squatting
with
dumbbells.

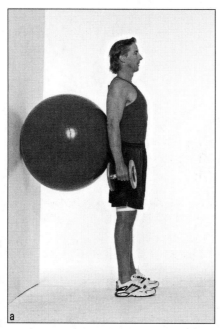 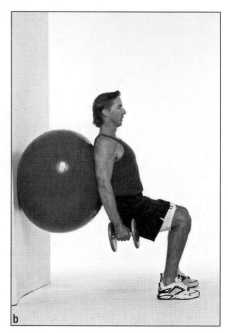

2. **Slowly squat down, keeping your knees bent at a 90-degree angle and your abdominal muscles tight and pulled in (see Figure 13-6b).**

   Your arms should remain relaxed at your sides.

3. **Hold this position for a few seconds and then slowly return to a standing position.**

Complete 10 to 15 repetitions.

A few do's and don'ts for this exercise:

✔ *Do* keep your knees in alignment with your toes. Never extend your knees past your toes.

✔ *Do* tighten your abdominal muscles to help keep your back strong and straight.

✔ *Don't* forget to press into the ball as you move into the squatting position. Doing so helps the ball roll along the wall and with your body.

Biceps curls on the ball

The instability of the ball and the heavier weight add new aspects to the classic biceps curl, making it more challenging.

To do this exercise, follow these steps:

1. **Sit on the ball with your feet shoulder-width apart. Hold your weights down by your sides with your palms facing inward.**

2. **Pull in your abdominal muscles as you slowly bring your weights toward your shoulders (see Figure 13-7).**

   Your palms will be facing your shoulders.

   Concentrate on the biceps muscles as you curl the weights toward your shoulders. This helps you isolate the movement and focus on the muscle that you're working.

3. **Hold the curl for a few beats and then release the weights back down to your sides.**

Complete two sets of 10 to 15 repetitions.

Here are a couple of do's and don'ts for this exercise:

✔ *Do* keep a straight spine while you're lifting the weights to your shoulders.

✔ *Do* lower the weights slowly back to starting position.

✔ *Don't* jerk the weights up to your shoulders. Use a small controlled movement instead.

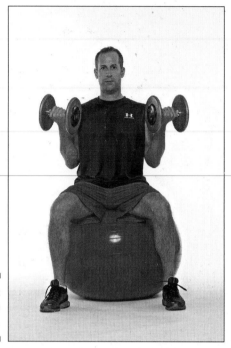

Figure 13-7:
Biceps
curls.

Alternating biceps curls on the ball

When doing alternating biceps curls, you may experience a subtle shifting of your weight on the ball, so you need to concentrate on maintaining your balance throughout this exercise.

To do this exercise, follow these steps:

1. **Sit on the ball with your feet shoulder-width apart. Hold your weights down by your sides with your palms facing inward.**

2. **Pull in your abdominal muscles as you slowly bring your right weight toward your right shoulder (see Figure 13-8).**

   Your palm will be facing in toward the shoulder.

3. **Hold the position for a few beats, and then release the weight back down to your right side and repeat with your other arm.**

Complete two sets of ten repetitions.

A few do's and don'ts for this exercise:

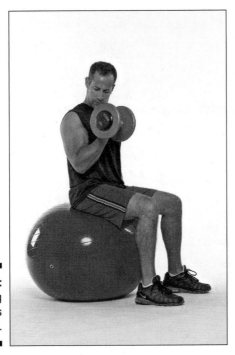

Figure 13-8:
Alternating
biceps
curls.

> ✔ *Do* concentrate on your biceps muscle as you do this exercise.
>
> ✔ *Do* contract your abs before lifting the weight to your shoulder.
>
> ✔ *Don't* jerk the weight up to your shoulder. Use a slow and controlled movement.

Ways to burn more fat

Besides building more muscle to burn fat, there are other good ways that you can get in shape and jump-start your metabolism. Here are a few things you can do throughout the day to make a difference:

✔ **Eat early in the day.** Most people try to go all day or at least a large portion of it without eating, thinking that this strategy will reduce their appetite and their caloric intake. Of course, you know what happens — you get extremely hungry because you waited too long to eat, so you eat more than you would have in the first place. And you don't have all day to burn it off the way you would have had if you'd eaten earlier. Remember, you actually boost your metabolism by eating a good breakfast (a break from fasting overnight) and you will feel better as you go about your day.

(continued)

(continued)

✔ **Exercise at night.** After sitting around all day, getting motivated to get off the couch and hit the gym or take a walk can be tough. But studies show that after doing a 60- to 90-minute workout in the evening, your metabolism is elevated 10 percent more the next morning. Now *that's* what we call burning calories in your sleep.

✔ **Refuel your body.** Keeping your body fulfilled or refueled every three to four hours with small healthy meals doesn't only give you more energy, but it also helps keep your weight down. Eating small meals throughout the day rather than three large meals stabilizes your blood-sugar levels, which helps your body burn fat more efficiently.

✔ **Take a jog or walk the dogs.** If you have big dogs like I do, taking a brisk walk or jog at night is great because their pulling motion really gets you going. If you don't have dogs, taking a 30-minute walk three to five times a week really makes a difference. Studies show that you actually burn the same amount of fat calories with a low-intensity 30-minute walk when done regularly as you would doing a 15-minute run for an equal distance.

Chapter 14

Easy Stretch Workout on the Ball

. . . .

. . . .

*I*n recent years, the ball has become a favorite of chiropractors and physical therapists because its round shape allows your body to stretch in a way that isn't possible using the floor or other devices. As the following stretches in this chapter demonstrate, draping your body over the ball is great for getting a good back stretch and for relaxing.

This chapter walks you through some amazing stretches that help you stretch your back and spine while you improve your flexibility like never before.

You can do the stretches in this chapter before you begin your regular workout, not only to get your circulation going, but also to help you gain coordination when working on the ball. Or, you can make stretching your entire workout if you're wanting to take things easy.

Benefits of Increasing Flexibility

Everybody's *flexibility,* or range of motion, differs because it's specific to individuals' joints. Some people can stretch like a rubber band, whereas others have a hard time touching the floor with their hands. Of course, the goal in all these stretches is to extend your range of motion so that everyday activities are easy and effortless.

Whatever group you fall into, here are a few of the benefits of increasing your flexibility:

- Stretching relieves lower back pain by elongating the key muscles that control the pelvic and back area, such as the hamstrings, lumbar muscles, hip flexors, and glutes.

- Stretching heats up the core muscles of your body, which makes performing all movements easier throughout the day.

- You expend less energy during a workout because of increased flexibility.

- Stretching reduces stress by increasing the blood supply to tight, tense muscles.

- Stretching gives you better posture by realigning and strengthening the muscles that support coordination and movement.

- Stretching reduces injuries because you have better control over your body's movements.

Starting with Upper Body Stretches

I always suggest working your body from the top and then downward because it warms up the body slowly and keeps you from getting dizzy, so I start this workout with some great stretches for your upper body.

Bending in all kinds of directions

Flexion, extension, abduction, adduction. All those terms sound kind of confusing when all you're really learning to do is bend! The truth is, when you bend your body in different ways, you gain the ability to work entirely different muscle groups. When you stretch muscles in opposition, you strengthen them and improve flexibility at the same time.

- *Flexion* is bending, or decreasing the angle, at the joint.

- *Extension* means straightening, or increasing the angle, at the joint. For instance, if you flex your foot, you work the front of your shin. If you extend your foot, you work the calf muscle in opposition.

- *Abduction* and *adduction* also work in opposition to each other and are terms best described as working your arms or legs toward the body or away from it.

If you bring your legs or arms toward, or into, your body, you're adducting them. If you take your arms away from your body, you're abducting them.

Whichever way you happen to be stretching, using slow, controlled movements gives you the best results and helps you achieve strength and flexibility at the same time.

Feel free to mix and match the following exercises any way you like. However, I find doing them in the following order works best because you get your blood flowing first before you jump into a full body stretch.

For the following stretch sequence, try using an exercise mat or a towel under your knees for comfort.

Shoulder stretch

The shoulder stretch stretches your chest muscles along with the muscles in front of your shoulder. You can stretch one shoulder at a time or both shoulders at once (as the following exercise shows).

To do this exercise, follow these easy steps:

1. **Kneel behind the ball and stretch your arms out in front of you (as Figure 14-1 shows).**

   Place only one arm on the ball for an individual stretch, and then alternate sides.

2. **Breathe out as you relax your body toward the floor, stretching your shoulder muscles.**

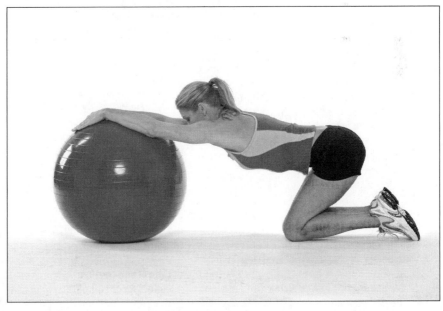

Figure 14-1:
Shoulder
stretch.

Hold the movement for a few seconds before you release back up. Repeat two or three times.

A few do's and don'ts for this exercise:

✔ *Do* allow your head and neck to relax toward the floor by casting your eyes downward.

✔ *Do* exhale with effort as you relax your body and stretch toward the floor.

✔ *Don't* let the ball move. Keep it steady and directly underneath your arms.

Upper back stretch

In this exercise, you feel a good stretch across your upper back as you let your upper body and arms drop toward the floor. This stretch is a great seated stretch that feels good to do right after the shoulder stretch.

To do this exercise, follow these steps:

1. **Sit on the ball with your back straight and your feet hip-width apart.**

2. **Lean forward from your waist as you wrap your hands under your lower legs and let your head relax down (as Figure 14-2 shows).**

Stretching techniques

Many medical conditions and groups of people, such as arthritis sufferers and fibromyalgia patients, are all good candidates for stretching on the ball. As with anything, you have to pace yourself, but the relief you gain from daily stretching sessions will provide you with a greater range of motion, which results in greater comfort.

You can use many different techniques to enhance your stretching, but here are the two most common:

✔ **Active stretching:** With this technique, you contract a muscle to put force on the opposite muscle that you're stretching. For example, if you extend your leg in front of you or rest it on a chair, you contract the quadriceps (the muscles that run along the front of your leg) while you stretch the

hamstrings (the muscles that run along the backside of your leg).

✔ **Passive stretching:** Passive stretching is when you apply an external force, such as your own body weight, bands, or free weights, to the muscle that you're stretching. For instance, if you lay your upper body over your leg as you extend it in front of you, you are using gravity and the force of your own body weight to stretch the leg.

Both stretching techniques are effective for increasing flexibility; however, passive stretching leads to more muscle development because of the external force or extra weight that you use. Active stretching is more common with athletes and people who need to develop muscle strength for particular activities that use both strength and coordination.

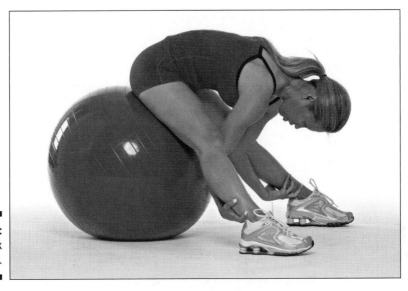

Figure 14-2:
Upper back
stretch.

3. **Gently pull with your arms to get a good stretch across your upper back.**

4. **Hold for a few seconds, and then release back up to your starting position and rest your hands on your thighs.**

A couple of do's and don'ts for this exercise:

✔ *Do* hold on to your shins or lower legs to get a good stretch through your upper back.

✔ *Don't* forget to exhale as you bend forward over your legs. Exhaling increases your stretch by allowing your body to relax farther toward the floor.

Side stretch

The *side stretch* targets the muscles that run along your waistline or your obliques. This exercise helps elongate your waist and stand taller.

To do this exercise, follow these steps:

1. **Kneeling on the floor next to the ball, rest your left side and left arm on the ball. Place your right palm on the back of your head (as Figure 14-3a shows).**

   You will be kneeling on your right knee as your rib cage is positioned against the ball.

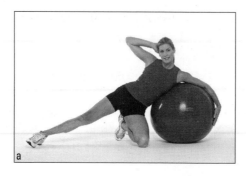

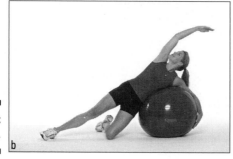

Figure 14-3:
Side stretch.

2. **Exhale as you raise your right arm over your head to stretch the left side of your body (see Figure 14-3b).**

3. **Inhale as you release your arm and side down to the starting position.**

Complete ten repetitions before you switch sides.

A few do's and don'ts for this exercise:

✔ *Do* place a towel or exercise mat under your knees for support.

✔ *Do* exhale before you extend your arm over your head.

✔ *Don't* forget to use the leg that you straightened to the side of your body as an anchor to keep the ball from moving.

Triceps stretch

This stretch is great for your triceps (the muscles that run along the back of your upper arms).

To avoid injury, do not pull on your elbow when you do this stretch.

To do this exercise, follow these simple steps:

1. **Sit on the ball with your feet shoulder-width apart. Reach your right arm toward the ceiling.**

2. **Bend your right arm at your elbow, bringing your right hand down to the back of your neck or between your shoulder blades (see Figure 14-4).**

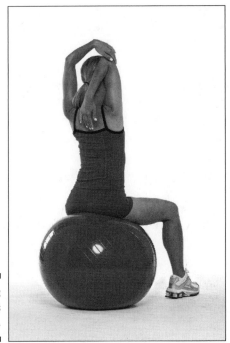

Figure 14-4:
Triceps
stretch.

3. **Using your left hand, gently stretch your elbow or upper arm downward.**

4. **Hold this stretch for a few seconds before you release your arm. Repeat on your other side.**

Complete three or four stretches on alternating sides.

A few do's and don'ts for this exercise:

✔ *Do* make sure that you feel a stretch on the back of your upper arm.

✔ *Do* keep your head up, not down, as you perform this stretch.

✔ *Don't* tug at your arm; instead, pull gently on the arm that you're stretching.

Neck stretch

You can always tell when someone has had a bad day or is stressed out because his shoulders are up next to his neck or he's complaining of a neck ache. Stretching out the muscles that lie alongside your neck and shoulders helps you release any built-up tensions in this area.

You can use your hand to pull gently downward as you stretch or just let the weight of your head do the stretch for you. Whichever way you choose to do this exercise, be sure not to pull or tug at your neck. Simply let the weight of your hand help your head and neck relax down and to the side.

To do this exercise, follow these steps:

1. **Sitting on the ball with your feet shoulder-width apart, relax your right ear to your right shoulder.**

2. **Gently place your right hand on your head or near your temple, letting the weight of your hand relax your neck and shoulders downward (as Figure 14-5 shows).**

   Let your left arm relax down the side of the ball as your right hand is on your head.

3. **Hold this stretch for a few seconds before you return to starting position and alternate sides.**

Complete three or four times on each side.

A few do's and don'ts for this exercise:

✔ *Do* roll your shoulders up and down between neck stretches to keep you loose.

✔ *Do* sit tall during this exercise and keep your back straight.

✔ *Don't* rush through this stretch. Take your time and breathe as you stretch the side of your neck muscles and your shoulders.

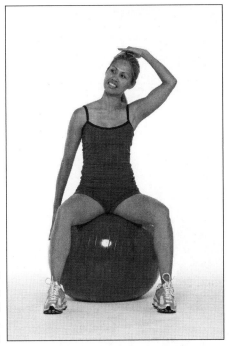

Figure 14-5:
Neck
stretch.

Oh, My Aching Back: Great Back Stretches

The following stretches balance your spine and stretch out your core. The drape stretch is my hands-down favorite, and it's likely to be yours, too. Even my soon-to-be 2-year-old loves it!

After doing the drape, the backbend stretch helps release your back and provides you with great flexibility in your lower back muscles.

The drape

The drape is a favorite of many chiropractors because it naturally stretches your back muscles using your own weight placed over the ball. Adding a gentle rock to the drape is soothing and gentle.

To do this exercise, follow these steps:

1. **Kneel behind the ball and rest your arms at your sides.**

2. **Drape your body over the ball face down, resting your fingertips and feet on the floor for support (as Figure 14-6 shows).**

   Let your head and neck relax to the floor.

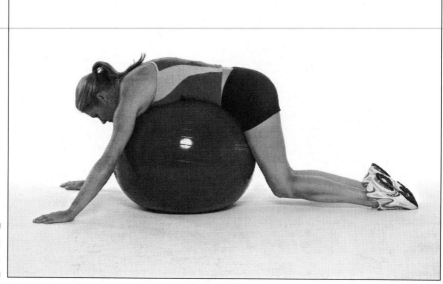

Figure 14-6:
The drape.

3. **Gently rock back and forth, releasing your back of any built-up tension or tight muscles.**

4. **Come back to starting position and rest on your knees before you repeat this stretch again.**

Repeat three to five times.

A couple of do's and don'ts for this exercise:

- ✔ *Do* let your body relax toward the floor during this exercise.

- ✔ *Don't* forget to breathe, which allows your back muscles to release farther toward the floor.

- ✔ *Don't* forget to let your head and neck hang down in a relaxed position.

Backbend stretch

In this stretch, you do a backbend, but it's a lot easier to do with the support of the ball. You also get a good stretch through your *trunk,* or your entire upper body, that leaves you feeling more open and relaxed than ever!

To do this exercise, follow these steps:

1. **Lie face up and drape your body over the ball, keeping your knees bent and your feet flat on the floor (as Figure 14-7a shows).**

   Your heels will be touching the floor.

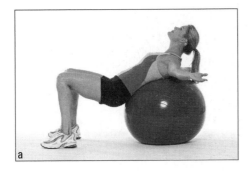

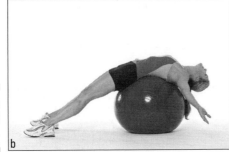

Figure 14-7: Backbend stretch.

2. **Open your arms out to your sides in an airplane position and extend your legs in front of you, rolling the ball out slightly (see Figure 14-7b).**

3. **Drop your hips and bend your knees to come back to starting position.**

Repeat five times, resting in between each repetition.

A couple of do's and don'ts for this exercise:

✔ *Do* keep your feet on the floor at all times.

✔ *Don't* forget to breathe as you lift up and back into this stretch.

Prone stretch

Lying face down on the ball is called being in the *prone position*. The prone position helps strengthen your upper and lower back muscles by training your stabilizing muscles (located along your spine). Having strong stabilizing muscles encourages good posture and better balance.

In other words, by raising your body off the ground and supporting your pelvis and spine, the prone position allows your body to move easily through a wider range of movements.

For this exercise and all exercises that originate in the prone position, place the ball under your lower abdomen and hips for support.

To do this exercise, follow these easy steps:

1. **Kneel behind the ball with your arms at your sides.**

2. **Roll your body forward onto the ball until your hips rest comfortably on top of it.**

3. **Place your hands on the ball for support (as Figure 14-8 shows).**

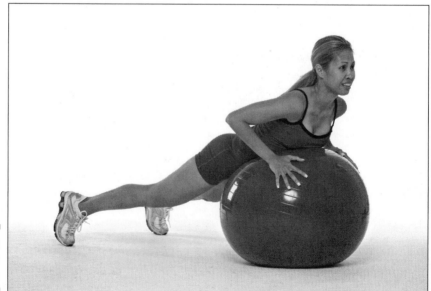

Figure 14-8:
Prone
position.

4. **Keeping the balls of your feet on the ground, raise your chest using your back muscles and not the strength of your arms.**

5. **Hold for a few seconds before releasing back to starting position.**

Complete five repetitions, resting between each one.

A few do's and don'ts for this exercise:

- ✔ *Do* keep your feet close together to help stabilize you on the ball.
- ✔ *Do* keep your eyes gazing down at the floor to keep your neck in line with your spine.
- ✔ *Don't* use your arms to lift your chest; instead, use your back muscles.
- ✔ *Don't* rush the movement.
- ✔ *Don't* forget to rest in between each lift.

Loosening Your Lower Half

The area that contains all the large muscle groups is the lower body. To create a leaner look in your lower half, try the hamstring stretch. To elongate your legs, try the following butt and back stretch.

You can do all the following lower body stretches at the end of your stretch workout or after a more intense full-body workout to help you cool down and stretch out your muscles.

Quads stretch

The quad stretch helps elongate and stretch your *quadriceps* (the muscles that run along the *front* of your upper leg). Most people who have tight quads usually also have tight *hamstrings* (the muscles that run along the *back* of the upper legs).

I suggest stretching your quadriceps first and then doing the following hamstring stretch to make sure that your entire leg is getting an even and balanced workout.

To do this exercise, follow these steps:

1. **Lie over the ball in prone position or with the ball under your hips and lower abdomen.**

2. **Keep your right arm and right leg on the floor as you lift your left leg behind you.**

3. **Raise your left arm up and reach behind you to grab onto your left ankle (as Figure 14-9 shows).**

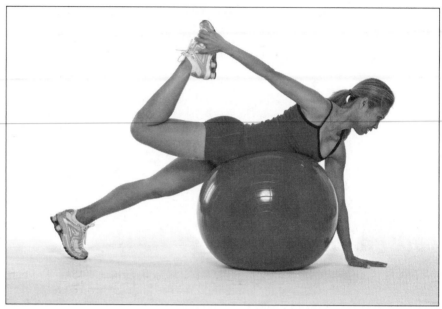

Figure 14-9:
Quads
stretch.

4. **Use a gentle lifting motion to lift up your left leg, stretching the front of your leg.**

5. **Hold this stretch for a few seconds before you lower your left arm and left leg to the floor.**

6. **Change arms and legs before repeating.**

Repeat five times on each leg, switching sides between repetitions.

A few do's and don'ts for this exercise:

✔ *Do* keep your supporting hand and foot slightly out to the side of the ball for added support.

✔ *Do* keep your eyes looking forward to avoid straining your neck and letting your head drop down.

✔ *Don't* push your ankle too far down so that it touches your butt. Gently pull your leg toward your butt to avoid placing any stress on your knee.

Hamstring stretch

This seated hamstring stretch is good to do right at your desk, especially if you've already replaced your desk chair with the ball. Tight hamstrings are a big problem for men and women because of all the sitting we do everyday. Try this stretch right after sitting on a hard chair, and you're sure to feel looser in no time!

To do this exercise, follow these steps:

1. **Sit with your weight forward on the ball and your feet more than shoulder-width apart.**

2. **Turn your body to one side and lean forward from your waist, lowering your chest toward your leg.**

   Let your hands rest on your upper leg for support or keep them on your hips.

3. **Roll the ball back slightly and extend your leg to one side until it's straight (as Figure 14-10 shows).**

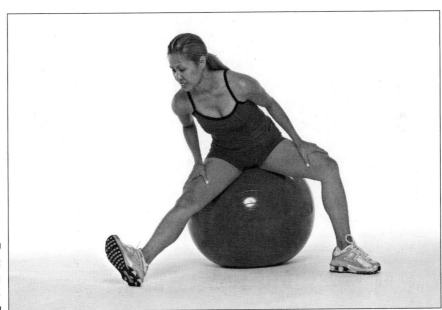

Figure 14-10:
Hamstring
stretch.

4. **Hold this position for a few seconds before you bend your knee and roll back up into starting position.**

5. **Repeat on the other side using your opposite arm and leg.**

Complete five stretches on each side.

A few do's and don'ts for this exercise:

✔ *Do* keep your back straight as you bend over your leg.

✔ *Do* bend your knee before you roll back up.

✔ *Don't* drop your head down. Keep your gaze straight ahead to avoid putting any strain on your neck.

Butt and back stretch

This exercise stretches out your back, butt, and hamstrings by rolling the ball behind you. The lower your upper body comes to the floor, the more stretch you get in the lower half of your body.

To do this exercise, follow these steps:

1. **With your feet wider than shoulder-width apart, sit with your weight forward on the ball.**

2. **Lean forward with your chest, keeping your back straight the entire time.**

3. **Place your hands on your upper legs or thighs (as Figure 14-11 shows).**

   Place your hands on the floor in front of you, if you feel you need an additional stretch.

4. **Slightly roll the ball behind you to increase the stretch in your butt, back, and legs.**

5. **After holding the stretch for a few seconds, roll your body back up into starting position.**

Complete five to ten repetitions.

A few do's and don'ts for this exercise:

✔ *Do* hold your stretch before rolling back up into starting position.

✔ *Do* widen your feet to get closer to the floor to intensify this stretch.

✔ *Don't* arch your back at all. Keep it straight and bend from your waist.

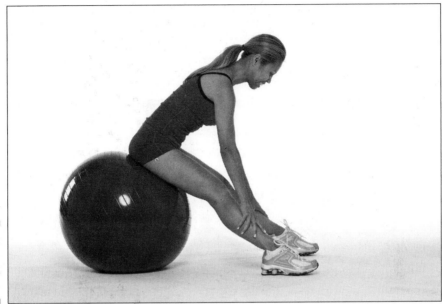

Figure 14-11:
Butt and
back
stretch.

Gluteal stretch

The gluteal stretch helps loosen your hips as well as your butt muscles, which are responsible for most of the important movements that you do throughout the day. Lower back pain can be a result of tight glutes, so stretching them out as often as possible is important!

To do this exercise, follow these steps:

1. **Lie on the floor with your feet on the ball and your knees bent at a 90-degree angle.**

2. **Place your ankle on your opposite thigh, letting the knee fall to the side (as Figure 14-12 shows).**

3. **Slightly roll the ball toward your body, increasing the stretch in your butt and hips.**

4. **After a few seconds, release your leg and foot down to the ball and repeat on your other side.**

Complete five times on each side.

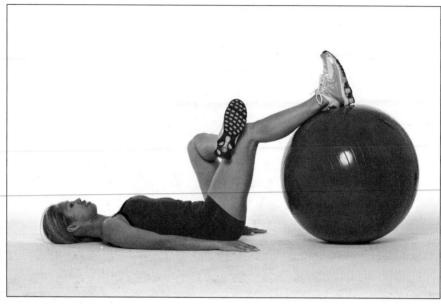

Figure 14-12: Gluteal stretch.

A couple of do's and don'ts for this exercise:

- ✔ *Do* let your knee fall to the side to get a good stretch in your lower body.
- ✔ *Don't* place your ankle on your knee; keep your ankle on your thigh to avoid any stress to your knee joint.

Reach and release

This stretch is a good one because it leaves you feeling taller and brings your body back to the floor.

Take a few good inhales and exhales as you extend your arms overhead to get an even better stretch from your fingertips to the end of your toes.

To do this exercise, follow these steps:

1. **Lie on the floor with your back in neutral spine and your legs straight out in front of you, making sure you point your toes.**

2. **Inhale as you place the ball over your head and stretch out with your arms as far as you can with the ball behind you (as Figure 14-13 shows).**

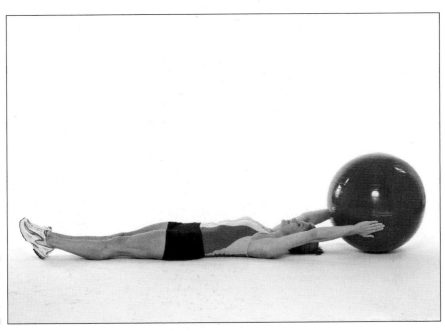

Figure 14-13:
Reach and
release.

3. **Exhale as you relax your arms farther behind your body.**

Complete five times.

A few do's and don'ts for this exercise:

✔ *Do* rest the ball on the floor behind you, not lifted off the ground.

✔ *Do* remember to breathe deeply during this exercise.

✔ *Don't* forget to point your toes, which gives you an extra stretch along the entire length of your body.

Chapter 15

Cardio and Go: Aerobic Exercise with the Ball

- -

In This Chapter

▶ Finding the right ball classes for you

▶ Knowing when you're burning fat

▶ Using ball exercises to get a cardio workout

▶ Performing ball exercises in different combinations

▶ Discovering ten-minute cardio workouts

- -

Can you really get a good cardiovascular workout on the ball? Can the workout really get your heart rate up and be as effective as a kickboxing class? You bet ya! Plus, getting your heart rate up and getting a great cardiovascular workout can be a lot more fun on the ball.

Doing the exercises in this chapter — and perhaps even adding a few small jumps in between — will raise your heart rate and help you work up a good old-fashioned sweat, just like any aerobics class. So have a ball!

Considering Ball Classes

Ball classes vary in technique and content quite a bit and depend on the individual instructor. Some classes incorporate resistance bands for a total body workout, or what's sometimes called a *ball and band class*. Some classes incorporate smaller medicine balls for added resistance (I cover medicine balls in Chapter 16).

Resistance classes using the ball work your muscles as never before by incorporating balance and stability. Because you can train and sculpt all the major muscle groups using the exercise ball, classes are a good way to work the same old muscles in a new, fun way. Working out on the ball in a class will also keep your heart rate up due to the pace and intensity that you'll get from the added resistance of weights, bands, or just the ball exercises themselves.

To find the right class for your level of fitness, check with the instructor before the class begins to see whether it's geared toward beginners or more experienced exercisers. Most beginning classes start out by using the ball in a warm-up to get your heart rate up, and then progress through a series of abdominal strengthening exercises and stretches. More advanced classes focus on using weights and other forms of resistance to increase the level of difficulty on the ball. When you've gained the balance and control you need to use the ball throughout a series of strengthening exercises, I suggest trying one of the more advanced classes that incorporates some additional equipment.

Making Sure You're Burning Fat

Can you still fit into your "skinny jeans"? You know, the ones that feel so good when you fit into them yet so bad when they're too tight? If you can't fit into your skinny jeans but you've been working out lately, then your body's telling you to try something new. If you're not working out and you can't fit into your skinny jeans, then you've already answered your question.

When you start working out, you ultimately gain muscle, and using a scale can be deceiving — not to mention discouraging — because muscle weighs more than fat (yep, the rumor's true, folks). But you need the muscle you gain to burn the fat into nice, lean muscle mass that actually weighs more than fat. So how can you tell your level of fitness and whether you're burning fat? Here are a few ways:

- ✔ **Get a heart rate monitor:** The first way to measure your fitness level is to use a heart rate monitor (see Chapter 5 for more info on this topic). A heart rate monitor measures your individual level of exertion and helps you train as close as possible to your maximum heart rate without going over, so you always know when you're in your fat-burning zone. To find your fat-burning zone, subtract your age from 220, and then multiply by 0.60 (or 60 percent) and 0.70 (or 70 percent). When you're using 60 to 70 percent of your maximum heart rate, you're burning 85 percent fat calories.

- ✔ **Check your pulse rate:** The second way to measure your fitness level is to take your pulse. To find your pulse rate, take a break in the middle of your workout when your heart rate is accelerated. Hold your index finger to your neck and count the beats per minute for 6 seconds. Take this number and add a zero to the end.

  For example, if your pulse rate were 14 beats in 6 seconds, after you add a zero to the end, your heart rate would be 140 for a full 60 seconds (one minute). This count gives you an accurate reading of your level of exertion.

Supersets: Training aerobically while you're lifting weights

Supersets are a way to train your body aerobically while pumping weights. Take two exercises that work a different body part — for instance, cycling and hand weights — and perform them one right after the other without resting in between or resting for no more than 30 to 45 seconds. This extra effort on your part gives you bigger gains and a smaller waistline because bigger muscles burn more fat!

To warm up your body, you should use 50 to 60 percent of your maximum heart rate. To train in your fat-burning zone, you should reach 60 to 70 percent of your maximum heart rate. And to train aerobically to strengthen your heart and improve your cardiovascular and respiratory systems, you should use 70 to 80 percent of your maximum heart rate.

✔ **Cross train:** To reach the next level of fitness, you can *cross train,* or use a combination of strength training along with aerobic training (some people call this *circuit training* because you move from one piece of equipment to another). I suggest warming up on the elliptical trainer for 10 minutes, strength-training with weights for 20 minutes, and ending with a 20-minute cool down on the treadmill.

Exercises for the Heart

The following exercises begin in a seated position on the ball to get your body moving and end with cardio bouncing in various cardio combinations.

Don't forget to take a moment to try one or all of these combinations and add some heart pumpin' music to make it more fun.

Heel touches

The object of this exercise is to keep the ball still as you reach out with your leg and alternate touching your heels to the floor. Believe me, this exercise isn't as easy as it looks!

To do this exercise, follow these steps:

1. **Sit tall on the ball with your feet shoulder-width apart and your hands at your sides.**

   Your hands will lightly touch the ball for support.

2. **Reach out with your right heel as you extend your right leg in front of you (see Figure 15-1).**

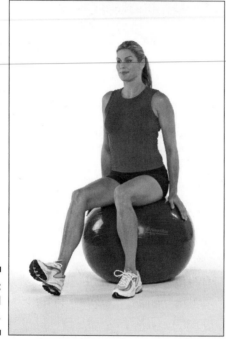

Figure 15-1: Heel touches.

3. **Return your right heel to starting position before you extend your left leg and heel to the opposite side.**

Alternate heel touches for two sets of 10 to 15 repetitions.

When you feel comfortable and balanced on the ball, try speeding up the movement.

A couple of do's and don'ts for this exercise:

   ✔ *Do* keep your back straight as you reach out and place your heel on the ground in front of you.

   ✔ *Don't* let your feet leave the ground at the same time. Always keep one foot on the floor.

Some ugly statistics

America is the fattest country in the world, and Americans spent $32 billion dollars last year alone on diet and weight-loss products. According to the U.S. Department of Health and Human Services, less than 10 percent of the population exercises three or more times a week at a level vigorous enough to improve cardiovascular fitness.

Marching

Marching is a fun exercise when done on the ball. The key to this exercise is to raise your knees as high as possible without losing your balance and falling backward off the ball.

To do this exercise, follow these steps:

1. **Sit tall on the ball with your feet shoulder-width apart and your hands at your sides.**

2. **As you tighten your stomach muscles for support, lift your right leg as high as possible (as Figure 15-2 shows).**

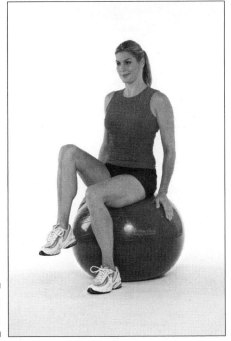

Figure 15-2:
Marching.

3. **Alternate lifting your legs in a marching fashion.**

   Continue marching for a few minutes until you've warmed up your hips.

A few do's and don'ts for this exercise:

  ✔ *Do* keep your knees pointed out in front, and not to the side, during this exercise.

  ✔ *Do* place your hands on the ball at either side of you for support.

  ✔ *Don't* let the ball move. Keep it as still as possible.

Side stepping

The side step opens up your pelvis and works your legs at the same time.

To keep from falling off the ball, sit up straight and maintain perfect posture.

To do this exercise, follow these steps:

1. **Sit tall on the ball and place your hands on either side of you.**

2. **Extend your right leg out and to the side, straightening your right knee (as Figure 15-3a shows).**

3. **Slowly bring in your right leg and extend your left leg out to the opposite side (see Figure 15-3b).**

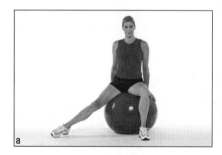

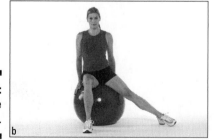

Figure 15-3: Side stepping.

Complete 15 repetitions on each side.

A few do's and don'ts for this exercise:

✔ *Do* keep your hands behind your body and on either side of you for support.

✔ *Do* straighten your leg as far as possible when you extend it to the side.

Side circles

In this exercise, you use a big sweeping motion to get your heart rate up quickly. Remember to warm up slowly and to use a controlled motion when swinging the ball from side to side.

The key to this exercise is to bend your legs slightly out to the sides, making room for the ball to move freely.

To do this exercise, follow these steps:

1. **Lift the ball above your head to start, and sweep the ball down to one side of your body (as Figure 15-4a shows).**

   Your body should remain loose so the ball can easily move while you keep your back straight for support.

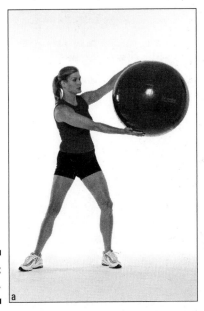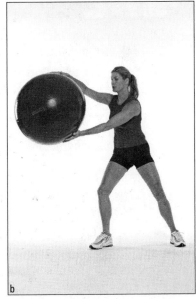

Figure 15-4:
Side circles.

2. **Sweep the ball down to the opposite side of your body as if you were swinging a pendulum from side to side (see Figure 15-4b).**

3. **Swing your arms and the ball back to your other side.**

Complete five repetitions of this exercise.

Some do's and don'ts for this exercise:

✔ *Do* keep a firm grip on the ball to keep it from flying out of your grasp.

✔ *Do* inhale and exhale while you swing your arms to help your body warm up more efficiently.

✔ *Don't* forget to bend your knees slightly as you move the ball from side to side.

Far-reaching ball squats

Far-reaching ball squats are great because they combine a squatting position with the extra weight of your upper body and the ball.

Make sure you get a wide enough stance with your legs so the ball can fit between your legs.

To do this exercise, follow these steps:

1. **Stand with your feet at least shoulder-width apart and hold the ball as far above your head as you can (as Figure 15-5a shows).**

2. **Using a squatting motion or bending your knees as you keep your back straight (refer to Figure 15-5b), lower the ball toward the floor.**

3. **Using your heels, press back up and straighten to standing position as you raise the ball back above your head.**

Complete five to ten repetitions.

A few do's and don'ts for this exercise:

✔ *Do* keep your back straight as you squat down with the ball.

✔ *Do* keep your gaze in the direction of the ball to keep from straining your neck.

✔ *Don't* let the ball touch the floor when you lower it.

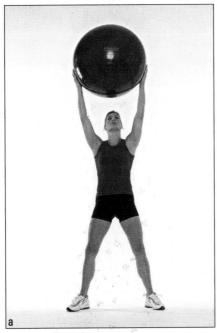

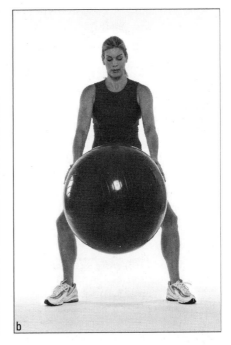

Figure15-5:
Far-
reaching
ball squats.

a

b

Side lunges

This exercise combines a lunging motion with a slight roll of the ball from side to side. You can do many cardio combinations with the ball just by adding a lunge that really can stretch out your *hamstrings* (the muscles that run along the back of your upper leg or thigh), your *quads* (the muscles that run along the front of your upper leg or thigh), and butt while increasing your heart rate.

Try adding a few far-reaching ball squats in between side lunges for a more intense warm-up.

To do this exercise, follow these steps:

1. **Bend one knee to the side in a lunge position and place the ball in front of your body within arm's reach.**

   Make sure that you use your opposite arm and leg when lunging; your back arm will rest on your thigh for support.

2. **Reach across your body with your arm and place your hand on the ball (as Figure 15-6 shows).**

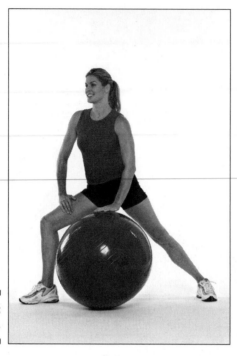

Figure 15-6:
Side lunges.

3. Lunge from side to side, rolling the ball to opposite sides of your body each time.

Complete ten repetitions.

A few do's and don'ts for this exercise:

- ✔ *Do* keep the ball in front of you at arm's length so you can control the ball as you roll it from side to side.
- ✔ *Do* reach out and across your body using your opposite arm and leg.
- ✔ *Don't* let your knee move beyond your toe as you lunge from side to side.

Side reaches

Side reaches stretch your *obliques,* or the side muscles that run along your rib cage, and help loosen the entire body and get the blood pumping in preparation for your workout.

To do this exercise, follow these steps:

1. **Sit tall and slightly forward on the ball.**

2. **Rolling the ball to the right, extend your left leg and reach your left arm over your head (as Figure 15-7 shows).**

   Keep your right hand on your thigh and your left leg bent to support your weight on the ball.

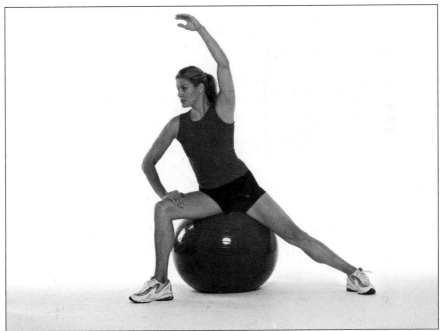

Figure 15-7:
Side reach.

3. **Lifting from your obliques (side muscles), straighten back up.**

4. **Repeat on the opposite side.**

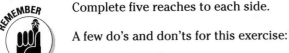

Complete five reaches to each side.

A few do's and don'ts for this exercise:

   ✔ *Do* sit slightly forward on the ball to make getting a complete stretch easier.

   ✔ *Don't* reach too far to the side because you can lose your balance.

   ✔ *Don't* forget to exhale as you reach to the side.

Cardio bouncing

Because the exercise ball doesn't have a handle to hold on to, you have to use your center of gravity and your hands to guide you as you do small bounces on the ball.

Remember that you're bouncing, not jumping. Be sure to keep your movements small.

Try placing the ball against a wall or a heavy object like a couch to keep the ball from moving when you jump up and come back down.

To do this exercise, follow these steps:

1. **Sit tall on the ball with your hands on either side of your body.**

2. **Using your legs, lift up and straighten your knees (as Figure 15-8a shows).**

3. **Return to starting position, being sure to replace your hands on either side of your body and back onto the ball for support (see Figure 15-8b).**

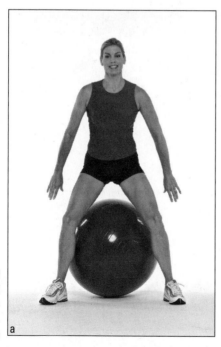
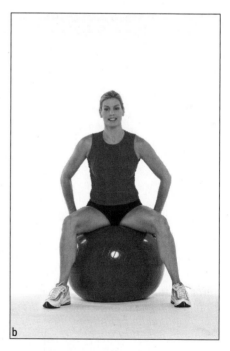

Figure 15-8: Cardio bouncing.

Grazing . . .

Eating every three hours or "grazing" all day is the best way to keep your body from storing fat. You need to maintain a steady amount of calories throughout the day to optimize your workouts and to keep up your energy. Counting calories or doing a program that emphasizes portion control is useful if you find eating throughout the day too overwhelming or if you just don't have the appetite.

Complete a series of 10 to 15 bounces before you rest and begin another set.

A couple of do's and don'ts for this exercise:

- ✔ *Do* use your leg and butt muscles rather than your hands to lift you off the ball.
- ✔ *Don't* go too far when you lift up; you're bouncing not jumping.

Ball Choreography and Sequences

You can create some really dynamic combinations using side lunges, far-reaching ball squats, side circles, and ball bouncing. Because these exercises are in a book and not demonstrated in a video, showing these combinations is harder to do. However, once you master the cardio exercises in this chapter, try putting them together as I do in the following choreography.

For the best way to get a great cardiovascular workout using the following choreography, try each combination two times before moving on to the next combination. After you've completed all five combinations in the following sequences, start over at the beginning or try mixing and matching the combinations if you've mastered them all!

Lunge combination

To do this sequence, follow these steps and do each step eight times:

1. **Stand and hold the ball out in front of your body, alternating touching your heels to the floor in front of you.**

2. **Step to the side and touch your opposite foot to your standing leg with the ball overhead.**

3. **With the ball on the floor in front of you, kick your leg right and lunge with your opposite leg to the left.**

4. **With the ball on the floor in front of you, punch with your right hand to the right and lunge to the side with your right leg; punch with your left hand to the left and lunge with your left leg to the left.**

A few do's and don'ts for this combination:

✔ *Do* keep the ball at chest level as you touch your heels in front of you or forward.

✔ *Do* kick slightly to the right or left side instead of straight forward to make room for the ball.

✔ *Don't* forget to repeat this combination several times before you move on to the next one.

Double lunge combination

To increase the challenge, add a small jump in between alternating lunges. Do each of the following steps eight times.

1. **Sitting on the ball, touch your heels one by one out in front of you — fast.**

2. **Sitting on the ball, slowly perform side steps.**

3. **Standing with the ball in front of you, perform alternating double lunges to the left and to the right.**

4. **Rolling the ball from side to side, alternate side reaches to the left and to the right.**

A couple of do's and don'ts for this combination:

✔ *Do* keep your hands on the ball for support while you're seated.

✔ *Don't* let your knee move beyond your toes when you perform a lunge.

Squatting combination

To do this sequence, follow these steps, performing each one eight times:

1. **Sitting on the ball, perform cardio bounces.**

2. **Standing with the ball overhead, do side circles.**

3. **Standing with the ball overhead, slowly do far-reaching ball squats.**

4. **Standing with the ball overhead, slowly do side circles with a squat in between.**

Some do's and don'ts for this combination:

- ✔ *Do* squat as if you were sitting down in a chair.
- ✔ *Do* challenge yourself by rising on your toes as you lift the ball above your head in the far-reaching ball squat.
- ✔ *Don't* forget to lunge from side to side for the side circles.

Step combination

A *grapevine* is a classic move or foot combination used with many aerobic combinations. It consists of stepping side, stepping back, and then stepping side again as you travel across the floor. Another way to describe the grapevine is as stepping front, stepping back, and then stepping front again as you move to the side.

To do this sequence, follow these steps:

1. **Hold the ball above your head and grapevine right and left four times.**
2. **Dribble the ball in front of you eight times or toss the ball above your head and catch it eight times.**
3. **Hold the ball out in front of your chest and grapevine right and left four times.**
4. **Dribble the ball to the side or toss and catch it eight times.**
5. **Side circle the ball eight times.**

A couple of do's and don'ts for this exercise:

- ✔ *Do* dribble the ball with alternating hands to test your agility.
- ✔ *Don't* forget to change arms each time on the grapevines.

Knee-touch combination

To do this sequence, follow these simple steps, doing each one eight times:

1. **Standing with the ball in your hands in front of your body, touch your knee to the ball.**
2. **Rolling the ball from side to side, alternate punching and lunging to opposite sides.**

3. **Standing with the ball in your hands in front of your body, touch your knee to the ball.**

4. **Rolling the ball from side to side, alternate kicking and lunging to opposite sides.**

A few do's and don'ts for this sequence:

✔ *Do* straighten your knee and leg as you kick to the front.

✔ *Do* touch the ball lightly to your knee so you don't knock it out of your hands.

✔ *Don't* forget to roll the ball slightly to the side as you lunge.

Quickies: Three Ten-Minute Cardio Workouts

Doing smaller ten-minute workouts called "time savers" twice a day or even just once a day is the new trend if you don't have an entire hour to work out. I guess that means the I-don't-have-time excuse won't be available to you anymore — we all have ten minutes! You can do these exercises on your lunch hour or before you wake up everyone in the house in the morning or even right after dinner instead of turning on the TV.

Here are a couple of ways to get a good old-fashioned workout in ten minutes (plus a few extra minutes for the warm-up and the cool down). You get the same results using these time-saver workouts twice a day as you do from doing a full hour of exercise because you get your heart rate up twice a day rather than once, which boosts your metabolism even more and helps you burn more calories.

Quickie #1: Jumping start

Grab a jump rope (and a towel for all your sweat!).

To do this ten-minute workout, follow these steps:

1. **Start with some jumping jacks to get your body warmed up and your heart pumping. Do these for about one minute.**

2. **Move on to lunges with the ball for three minutes (shown earlier in this chapter).**

3. **Jump rope for three minutes.**

4. **Get on the floor and do push-ups for one minute.**

5. **Stay on the floor and try some abdominal crunches on the ball for two minutes.**

6. **Cool down for three to five minutes. Start by walking at a fast pace and gradually slow your pace. As you come to a stop, end with a few stretches on the ball (hamstrings, quads, glutes), as Chapter 14 shows.**

The times that I include in these workouts are merely suggestions. Do only as many repetitions as you can while maintaining proper form. When you can't maintain proper form anymore, move on to the next exercise.

Quickie #2: Core combo

You need your ball and 3- to 5-pound hand weights for this series.

To do this ten-minute workout, follow these steps:

Start with one minute of jumping jacks to warm up your body and get your heart rate up.

1. **Using the ball, do the seated shoulder press (see Chapter 6).**

   Do 10 to 15 repetitions for each set, doing enough sets to total three minutes.

2. **Move on to the seated lateral arm raises (see Chapter 6).**

   Again, do 10 to 15 reps for each set, with enough sets to total three minutes.

3. **Drop your weights and lie with your tummy on the ball, alternating arm and leg raises (see Chapter 8) for one minute.**

4. **To work your abs, do some crunches on the ball (see Chapter 8) for two minutes.**

5. **To finish up, cool down for three to five minutes. Walk at a fast pace, gradually slowing your pace as you go. As you come to a stop, end with a few stretches on the ball (hamstrings, quads, glutes) as Chapter 14 shows.**

Quick picks: Weekly workout

Here's a complete workout plan that covers you for an entire week if you just pick four from the following list.

Got rest? The connection between sleep and heart disease

Studies have linked heart disease to smoking, high blood pressure, being overweight, and all those other things we know are bad for us, but what about sleep? New evidence suggests that not getting enough sleep or being sleep deprived can actually cause heart problems.

That link makes sense, if you think about it. When you don't get enough sleep or you sleep less than six or seven hours, it affects all your body's functions. Because your blood pressure is lower when you sleep, being awake for longer periods of time results in higher blood pressure. When your blood pressure is higher, your heart has to work harder to pump the blood through your body and places stress on your entire system.

Another negative effect of being sleep deprived is that your body releases higher levels of the stress hormone cortisol, which puts additional stress on your heart.

So what about people who sleep too long? Studies show that people who sleep more than nine or ten hours tend to be less active. They exercise less, drink more alcohol, tend to smoke, and weigh more than their counterparts (which isn't good for your heart).

Getting the proper amount of rest these days seems to be a bigger issue than just being plain tired or trying to find the time — it seems to be a matter of staying heart healthy. Here are a few suggestions for getting a healthier night's sleep:

✔ **Keep a regular bedtime and stick with it.** Going to bed at the same time every night sets your internal body clock so you can get a better night's rest; plus, your body knows what to expect.

✔ **Get a good workout.** People who exercise every day or at least a few times a week have a lot more energy during the day and sleep more soundly at night.

✔ **Play a relaxing tape or soothing music.** Studies show that the brain responds well to waterfall sounds or light music, which can help you drift off to sleep. In other words, turn off the TV! TV activates your brain and can keep you up longer than you'd like to be.

✔ **Read a good book.** Reading is a great way to put you to sleep. (It works for me every time!) Maybe you'll take this book to bed with you to fall asleep. Hmmm . . . is that a good thing?

✔ **Drink herbal or chamomile tea.** Some great blends of herbal teas can help you wind down and nod off quicker. I suggest trying chamomile tea.

Whatever you choose to do, remember that sleep is just as important an element in your life as exercise, so get your rest!

Always do a warm-up to increase your heart rate gradually and cool down properly when performing any of the following workouts.

- ✔ **Day One:** Warm up with the ball (see Chapter 5) then jump rope for 5 minutes.

- ✔ **Day Two:** Walk 3 miles. After cooling down properly, end with a few ball stretches (see Chapter 14).

- ✔ **Day Three:** Off!

- ✔ **Day Four:** Take a one-hour class at the gym; try a ball class, a spinning class, a core mat class, a step class, or a kickboxing class.

- ✔ **Day Five:** Perform the cardio exercises in this chapter and then jump rope for 5 minutes.

- ✔ **Day Six:** Off!

- ✔ **Day Seven:** Walk 2 miles. After cooling down properly, end with a few ball stretches (see Chapter 14).

You can switch up the days or save a few for the weekends. Just be sure you do all four!

Chapter 16

Adding Accessories to Your Workout on the Ball

· ·

In This Chapter

▶ Getting fit using resistance bands with the ball

▶ Knowing the difference between a medicine ball and a stability ball

▶ Getting a workout with two balls

▶ Performing upper and lower body exercises with accessories

▶ Discovering your level of resistance

· ·

*W*orking out on an exercise ball is definitely fun and effective, but when you use accessories, such as resistance bands or a medicine ball, your workout becomes more exciting and definitely more challenging. Adding accessories to your exercise ball workout not only increases your coordination, balance, and strength, but it also tones your entire body.

In this chapter, I give you the lowdown on these two handy accessories, and I cover upper and lower body exercises that you can do with these pieces of equipment. When used in conjunction with the exercise ball, they increase strength and assist in stretching the major muscle groups throughout the entire body.

One of the many advantages of using resistance bands instead of weights in your workout is that they're less intimidating than dumbbells and are much more versatile. Medicine balls also provide a great alternative to using weights because they feel more natural in your hand and are easy and fun to use.

Getting to Know Resistance Bands and Medicine Balls

Simply put, a *resistance band* is a piece of rubber tubing that provides resistance when you pull it — sort of like an oversized rubber band. Resistance bands range from a little resistance to a lot, and the band's color designates its level of resistance. Read on to find out which one band is the right one for you.

Medicine balls are similar in shape to a basketball and are used for training athletes in sports-specific exercises. These balls also come in different increments of weight to provide a strength-conditioning alternative to dumbbells and hand weights. Medicine balls provide a new way for you to increase your muscle tone and improve your posture when you combine them with the exercise ball. Check the following list to see where you need to start when you have your new accessories in hand.

Banding together

What makes this stretchy band so desirable to use while working out is its versatility. You can use it with a chair, under your feet, tied to a door, or under the ball. And when you compare it to weights or dumbbells, a resistance band is a go-anywhere alternative and it's much less expensive, costing around $1.40 per tube.

Resistance bands come in six to eight levels of resistance, which are identified by color. The three most-common levels are the

- ✔ **Yellow band:** The yellow band is light in resistance. It's commonly used by first-timers and usually ranges in resistance from 5 to 10 pounds.

- ✔ **Green band:** The green band is medium in resistance. This band is the most-commonly used and ranges in resistance from 10 to 15 pounds.

- ✔ **Red band:** The red band is heavy in resistance. Mostly advanced men and women use this band, which ranges in resistance from 15 to 25 pounds.

I recommend starting with a yellow band (the one with the least resistance) to give yourself the best chance at getting acquainted with using bands. As you gain more proficiency with the exercises on the ball, you can gradually increase your level of resistance.

Take your medicine

The medicine ball is a unique tool used for training athletes for sports-specific exercises. For instance, boxers, tennis players, and other professional athletes train using medicine balls. The medicine ball is superior to using weight machines that are bolted to the wall or floor because they provide resistance that gives you a full range of motion.

The medicine ball has been in use for years in Europe but has only recently gained popularity in America. The medicine ball, popular for its non-slip surface and full range of motion, found its way to the states through chiropractors and physical therapists who used them to strengthen patients' upper bodies and core muscles.

Combined with the exercise ball, the medicine ball becomes an amazing tool for a complete body workout. You can use it to strengthen your back, shoulders, arms, and legs as well as to strengthen your entire core (torso).

Medicine balls are always somewhat smaller than basketballs, but they come in different weights designated by different colors (just like resistance bands). The following is a list of the most popular colors and weights:

- Yellow: 2.2 pounds
- Green: 4.4 pounds
- Blue: 6.6 pounds
- Orange: 8.8 pounds
- Red: 11 pounds
- Yellow: 13.2 pounds
- Black: 15.4 pounds
- Green: 17.6 pounds

I recommend starting out with either the green 4.4-pound medicine ball or the blue 6.6-pound medicine ball before you graduate to a heavier weight. When combined with the exercise ball, a lower-weight medicine ball makes gaining the coordination you need to keep your balance on the ball while using added resistance easier.

Working Your Upper Body with the Ball and Band

The exercise ball makes a great partner for using the medicine ball and the band to tighten and tone your upper body. The following exercises use all three together to work your upper body.

Chest press

This exercise works your entire chest area — especially your pectoral muscles. It greatly defines your shoulders and back as well.

To do this exercise, follow these steps:

1. **Place the resistance band under the ball and lie with your upper back on the ball. Hold the handles or ends of the band in each hand (as Figure 16-1a shows).**

   Draw your navel to your spine to engage your abdominal muscles.

   Keep your legs directly under your knees at a 90-degree angle.

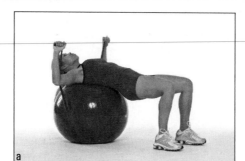

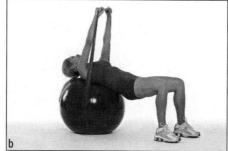

Figure 16-1: Chest press with resistance band.

2. **With your elbows bent to the sides and with your shoulders, press your hands to the ceiling as you contract the muscles in your chest (see Figure 16-1b).**

3. **Reverse this movement by relaxing your elbows back to your body and even with your shoulders.**

Complete two sets of ten presses, resting between sets.

Here are some do's and don'ts for this exercise:

✔ *Do* face your palms toward the ceiling as you press up. Your hands should face the wall in front of you.

✔ *Don't* let the ball move. Keep it still by supporting it with your legs and upper back.

Lat pulls

This exercise works the muscles that are located just above the rib cage and along the sides of the body.

To do this exercise, follow these steps:

1. **Sit on the ball with your feet shoulder-width apart. Begin with your arms up, holding the resistance band toward the middle and extending it overhead (as Figure 16-2a shows).**

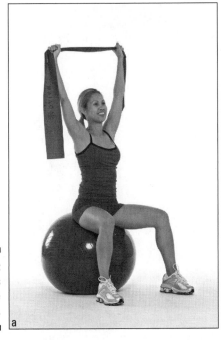 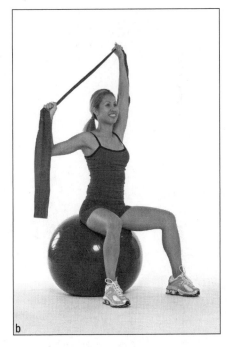

Figure 16-2: Lat pulls with the band.

a

b

2. **Bring your hands slightly close together before beginning, and then pull your arms out and down, bringing your elbows close to your rib cage (see Figure 16-2b).**

3. **Raise your arms back above your head and repeat, bring arms down to your other side.**

Complete two sets of ten reps on each side.

A couple of do's and don'ts for this exercise:

✔ *Do* sit tall and contract your stomach muscles.

✔ *Don't* rush through this exercise. Be sure to hold the band to the side for a few beats before returning to starting position.

Rear delts

This exercise works the back of your shoulders most commonly referred to as your shoulder blades.

To do this exercise, follow these steps:

1. **Sit on the ball with your feet shoulder-width apart. Hold the resistance band in the middle and extend your arms in front of you (as Figure 16-3a shows).**

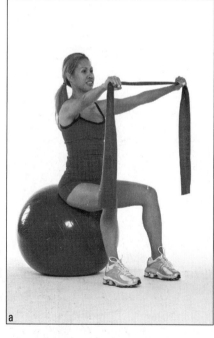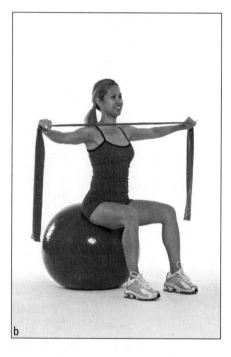

Figure 16-3:
Rear delts with the band.

a   b

2. **Squeeze your shoulder blades together and pull your arms out to the sides like an airplane (see Figure 16-3b).**

3. **Keeping tension on the band, return your arms to the starting position.**

Complete two sets of ten repetitions.

A couple of do's and don'ts for this exercise:

✔ *Do* hold the band in the middle to increase the difficulty.

✔ *Don't* release the band at any time. Keep tension on the band throughout the exercise.

Overhead press

Overhead press works the top of your shoulders and is also great for working your biceps.

To do this exercise, follow these steps:

1. **Sit on the ball with your feet shoulder-width apart, placing the resistance band under the ball. Bend your arms, keeping your elbows at shoulder level (see Figure 16-4a).**

   Your palms should be facing out.

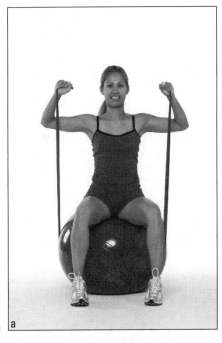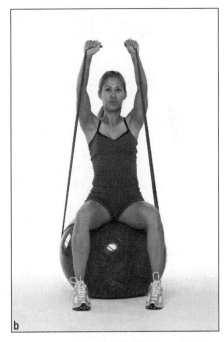

Figure 16-4: Overhead press with the band.

2. **Straighten your arms above your head and hold for a few seconds (as Figure 16-4b shows).**

3. Slowly bring your arms back to the starting position.

Complete two sets of ten repetitions.

Here are some do's and don'ts for this exercise:

✔ *Do* keep your wrists straight as you push your arms above your head.

✔ *Do* contract your abdominal muscles before pressing up.

✔ *Don't* lift your bottom off the ball. Keep it pressed down and steady.

Working Your Lower Body with the Ball and Band

The lower body really benefits from a workout that combines the band with the ball. Using these pieces of equipment together makes targeting the hamstrings, quadriceps, and gluteals all at once easier.

Bridge with leg extension

This exercise not only targets the quadriceps, but it also calls upon the abdominal muscles to keep the ball stable.

To do this exercise, follow these steps:

1. **Tie a knot in the band so that it's a little taut when you place it around your feet. Place the band around one ankle and under your other foot. Lie with your upper back on the ball in a bridge position (as Figure 16-5a shows).**

2. **As you tighten your stomach muscles, slowly lift one leg, pulling the band until your leg is straight (see Figure 16-5b).**

3. **Hold this position for a few seconds, and then return the leg to the starting position.**

Complete five lifts on each leg.

A couple of do's and don'ts for this exercise:

✔ *Do* extend your leg until the knee is straight.

✔ *Don't* arch your back.

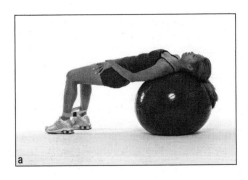

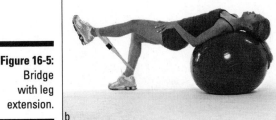

Figure 16-5:
Bridge
with leg
extension.

Plie with a band

A *plie* is a traditional ballet move that has become a common move in regular forms of exercise. Don't worry if you have two left feet — I tell you how to perform a proper plie so you can easily incorporate it into your exercise routine.

Performing this move gives your legs a long, sleek look, just like a dancer. Here's how you do it:

1. **Standing with your legs shoulder-width apart, turn your feet out to a 45-degree angle and descend toward the ground while opening your legs (this move works the inner thigh muscles, or the *adductors*) and keeping your butt tucked under your torso.**

2. **Continue to lower your butt toward the ground until it comes near the level of your knees.**

Try not to let your knees bend beyond your toes because you'll place too much stress on the knee itself. If you find yourself bending beyond this point, open your legs out farther, keeping your torso upright and trying not to let your chest drop forward.

Now that you have the plie down, you can try the plie with a band exercise. This exercise works your inner and outer thighs plus your lower back and gluteal muscles — otherwise known as your butt!

To do this exercise, follow these steps:

1. **Tie a knot in the band so that it's a little taut when you place it around your ankles (keep your ankles shoulder-width apart). Position the ball between you and the wall, resting your upper back on the ball and pointing your feet out to a 45-degree ankle (see Figure 16-6a).**

Figure 16-6:
Plies with a band.

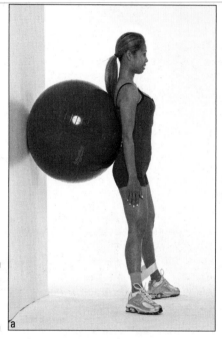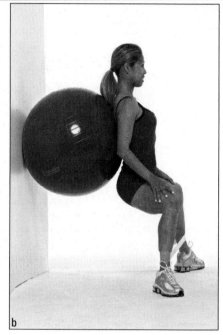

2. **Roll the ball down the wall, bending your knees to lower yourself until your thighs are parallel with the floor (see Figure 16-6b).**

3. **Press back up to the starting position, rolling the ball back up the wall.**

Complete 15 repetitions.

A couple of do's and don'ts for this exercise:

✔ *Do* keep your abdominal muscles tight and your back straight as you lower yourself toward the floor.

✔ *Do* press up with your inner thigh muscles.

✔ *Don't* let your knees extend out over your toes when pressing down into a plie.

Combining Your Exercise Ball with a Medicine Ball

I really like this next group of exercises that combine the medicine ball with the exercise ball because you can really develop some rock-hard abs and a trim waist by doing them. You'll find it helps strengthen your entire body from the added weight and resistance of the medicine ball. Good luck!

Crunches with medicine ball

This exercise works your *obliques,* or side muscles, that run along your waist.

To do this exercise, follow these steps:

1. **Lie face up with your upper back resting on the ball and your legs at a 90-degree angle. Extend your arms above your body, holding the medicine ball in both hands (see Figure 16-7a).**

   Draw your navel in toward your spine to engage your abdominal muscles.

2. **Lifting your upper back, contract your stomach muscles as you twist your body to the left, bringing the medicine ball and your arms toward your left thigh (see Figure 16-7b).**

3. **Lower back to starting position, bringing your arms back behind your head.**

Complete 15 repetitions, alternating sides.

A couple of do's and don'ts for this exercise:

✔ *Do* contract your abdominal muscles when you're lifting up your body.

✔ *Don't* reach too far to the side when you're twisting your body up. Go only as far as your outer thigh.

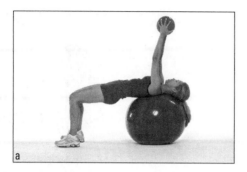

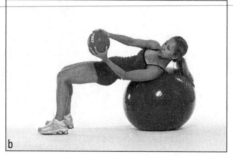

Figure 16-7:
Crunches
with a
medicine
ball.

Chest squeeze with medicine ball

Because of the twisting motion used in this exercise, your waist gets a work-out along with the pectoral muscles in your chest.

To do this exercise, follow these steps:

1. **Sit on the ball with your feet shoulder-width apart. Hold the medicine ball at chest level and squeeze, contracting your chest muscles (as Figure 16-8a shows).**

2. **Still squeezing the ball, twist your body to the left and push the ball out just a few inches (see Figure 16-8b).**

3. **Bring the ball back in and return your body to center, still squeezing the ball.**

Repeat the exercise on the other side. Complete 15 twists.

A couple of do's and don'ts for this exercise:

✔ *Do* keep your back straight and your abs tight during this exercise.

✔ *Don't* stop squeezing the ball at any time.

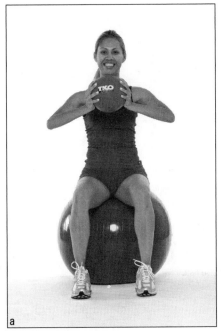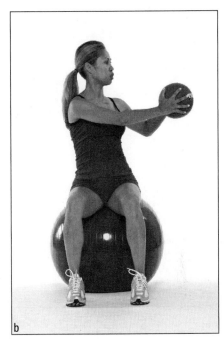

Figure 16-8:
Chest
squeeze.

a   b

Ball balance

This exercise may seem like a circus trick, but it's really just a good old test in balance and control.

If balancing on two balls proves too challenging, try pushing the exercise ball against a wall or a heavy couch for support.

To do this exercise, follow these steps:

1. **Sit on the exercise ball with your arms extended to the sides in an airplane position and rest one foot on the medicine ball (as Figure 16-9 shows).**

2. **When you have your balance, lift your other foot off the floor and place it on top of the medicine ball next to the existing foot.**

3. **Hold this position for ten seconds, and then release your foot back to the ground and repeat.**

Complete ten repetitions.

A couple of do's and don'ts for this exercise:

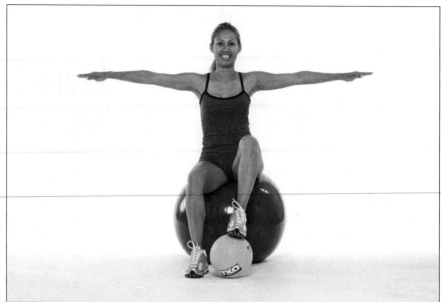

Figure 16-9:
Ball
balance.

✔ *Do* maintain a straight and long spine during this exercise.

✔ *Do* use your arms for balance.

✔ *Don't* start lifting your foot until you feel completely stable.

Chapter 17

Bending Over Backward: Yoga on the Ball

· ·

In This Chapter

▶ The nuts and bolts of yoga

▶ Knowing the benefits of doing yoga with the ball

▶ Trying a few basic yoga on-the-ball exercises

· ·

*I*n the past few years, yoga has grown tremendously as an acceptable and desirable form of exercise. Everyone from athletes to celebrities just can't enough of it. When you combine it with the exercise ball, yoga becomes the perfect combination of balance and strength. Many challenging yoga poses become easier by supporting your body weight with the ball.

In this chapter, I cover several traditional yoga moves adapted specifically for use on the ball. You can incorporate the exercises in this chapter into your regular workout, use them as part of your stretch program on the ball (see Chapter 14), or use them at the end of your cardiovascular workout on the ball (see Chapter 5) or off. If you really get into using yoga postures combined with the ball, I recommend reading *Yoga on the Ball* by Carol Mitchell (Healing Arts Press), where you can get a complete understanding of how to combine traditional yoga postures with the exercise ball.

Basic Principles of Yoga

Yoga is an Eastern discipline used to move the energy throughout your body. The more freely the energy flows, the more energetic you feel. Practicing yoga is meant to help bring your life into a state of balance and composure.

Using yoga as a form of exercise is a Western approach (and what I describe in this chapter) that deals strictly with the physical body. By keeping your body relaxed and loose using stretching poses executed in a series of movements, yoga can help reduce years of wear and tear.

Expanding your mind

Some people call yoga "awareness training" because it teaches you not to focus on where you are, how you're feeling, or where you're going, but to focus on being in the moment. As you do the workout in this chapter, try to think only of the movements and the positioning of your body on the ball. Then you will be in a true yoga state of mind.

Breathing deeply, really deeply

One of the primary principles of yoga is breathing. Focusing on your breath and letting it move you through any pain that has built up in your body is just as important as the yoga poses themselves. This exercise helps you locate any tension that has built up in your body and keeps your breath moving freely to supply oxygen to your heart, lungs, and throughout your body.

Here are a few steps for taking a good yoga breath:

Always breathe in and out through your nose, not your mouth.

1. **Lie flat on your back.**
2. **Begin by breathing slowly and deeply.**
3. **Let your stomach rise as it fills with air.**
4. **When your stomach fills with air and you feel that there's no more room, let your rib cage expand sideways.**
5. **Hold your breath for a few seconds.**
6. **Empty your lungs by relaxing your stomach and allowing your breath to flow.**

To ensure that you're breathing properly, place one hand on your stomach next to your belly button and feel your abdomen rise with air as you breathe. As you inhale deeper, place your other hand on the side of your rib cage to feel it expand even more.

Feeling the flow

Would you put a period at the beginning of a sentence? I doubt it. And for the same reason, the sequence of exercises in yoga is important. Flowing from one exercise to another lets your body warm up slowly and allows your mind to become attuned to what's going on in your body. This principle holds true for all forms of exercise because warming up your body first is always a good idea.

Benefits of Doing Yoga on the Ball

Many people know the toning benefits that yoga offers, and they also know the strengthening benefits of using the ball. But most people don't know or haven't tried combining the two, which provides both results at the same time by using the resistance of their own body weight. To really tone your muscles and strengthen your core, combining the ball with yoga is the way to go. Read on to find out more benefits of combining the ball with yoga.

Better balance

In everyday life, we do many simple movements that require good balance, a stable back, and strong abdominal muscles. A few examples are standing on a chair, reaching for a box of cereal, or bending over to do gardening work. Maintaining balance and flexibility are important to all these daily functions and are just a few of the key benefits you get when training on the ball with yoga.

When your abdominal muscles are weak, holding yoga poses for very long is difficult to do. The same is true when your back muscles are weak — everything else is weak, too. The ball helps you do yoga poses by supporting your body weight and allowing you to stretch your muscles in positions that you may not be able to without the support of the ball. For example, someone with a history of knee problems can use the ball to provide a stable base so she can stretch her knee and the surrounding muscles. For a pregnant woman, the ball can help her find the balance she desperately needs to offset her pregnant tummy. The ball can also help an older person find the balance he may have lost due to a sedentary lifestyle.

So, as you can see, training your stabilizing muscles (your abs and back muscles) with yoga poses on the ball can help prevent everyday injuries and possible accidents that you may otherwise have been susceptible to.

Better posture

Many people are replacing their chairs with the ball because sitting on the ball's uneven surface forces them to have good posture by making them engage their stabilizing muscles (the ones that lie deep within your body to support you as you sit up on the ball). When you combine yoga with the ball, you get the added benefit of stretching the muscles through the yoga postures and strengthening the spine by using the ball. Hence, you create good posture and strong alignment of the spine.

Most popular yoga styles

You can practice many different styles of yoga today, all of which originated from *hatha yoga,* or the Western form, which is physical in nature. "Hatha" means "sun" and "moon," which imply balance (because they're polar opposites), just as "yin" and "yang" implies balance. Practicing hatha yoga is intended to teach you to have control over your body and how your awareness and control relates to your everyday life.

Here are the more popular Western yoga styles rooted in hatha yoga:

- ✔ **Bikram:** This style of yoga is practiced in a 90- to 100-degree room in order to create steam or heat from the exertion of the yoga poses. This style has 26 poses that you always do in the same order.

- ✔ **Ashtanga:** Sometimes called "power yoga," ashtanga always begins with the sun salutation pose (which is one of the exercises I show you in this chapter) and synchronizes yoga poses with your breathing to help you flow through a series of movements.

- ✔ **Iyengar:** This style of yoga emphasizes poses that you hold much longer than the previous forms I listed. This style is a very intense workout or discipline that emphasizes symmetry, alignment, and precision.

- ✔ **Kundalini:** In this style of yoga, you incorporate chanting throughout a series of yoga poses. Through breathing, chanting, and movement, kundalini yoga awakens the energy that's stored at the base of your spine, which is known as *kundalini energy.*

- ✔ **Viniyoga or vinyasa:** This style of yoga is a more gentle style that's great for beginners because you learn it at a slower pace. A series of *vinyasa,* or flowing movements, coordinate with your breathing and the individual needs of each student.

- ✔ **Tantra:** This style of yoga integrates sexuality with spirituality. Through visualization, chanting, yoga poses, and breathing exercises, tantra yoga focuses the kundalini energy within your body and develops this energy or directs it for a greater sexual experience.

- ✔ **Yin:** This style of yoga works with the connective tissue and joints in your body rather than the primary muscles that other yoga forms use, which are known as the *yang* tissues and muscles. Yin yoga uses fewer poses than other forms of yoga and requires you to hold each pose for a longer period of time to allow your joints and the tight areas in your body to open up.

Whatever style of yoga you choose, you should always practice under the guidance of a qualified teacher because yoga is so individualized. Always make sure that you start at a beginning level before you progress into power yoga or a more vigorous form.

Warming Up Using Yoga on the Ball

Focus and breathing are essential to practicing yoga. The following exercises are great for reducing stress and calming your body and mind. You can also use them as part of your warm-up and cool down for your regular workout.

Yoga breathing with the ball

You can use the exercise ball to make yourself aware of the area you're using to breathe. To take a good yoga breath that's free of any tension and pain, you have to know where your breath is coming from. To help you locate and calm your breathing use your hand to feel your abdomen and rib cage rise.

To do this exercise, follow these steps:

1. **Lie on your back and bend your knees, keeping your feet flat on the floor.**

2. **Rest the ball on your abdomen and against your knees. Support the ball with your hands on either side (as Figure 17-1 shows).**

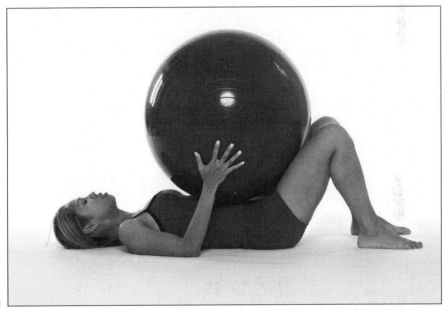

Figure 17-1:
Yoga
breathing
with the
ball.

3. **Take a deep breath, allowing the ball to rise as your belly fills with air.**

Inhale to the count of ten and exhale to the count of ten for several breaths.

Sun salutation

Sun salutation is a series of movements you do sequentially to warm up your body. Whether you do this exercise on the ball or standing, sun salutation always follows the same steps.

Don't forget to use your belly breathing throughout this exercise to help you flow through the stretch.

To do this exercise, follow these steps:

1. **Sit tall on the ball with your feet shoulder-width apart. Inhale as you bring your arms together above your head, clasping your hands together in a prayer position (as Figure 17-2a shows).**

2. **As you exhale, bend forward from your waist, touching your hands to your ankles (see Figure 17-2b).**

3. **Extend your right leg back in a lunge position and support your body weight by bringing your hands to the floor on either side of your front leg (as Figure 17-2c shows).**

4. **Lift your body back up by placing your hands on your front knee for support and then continuing to bring your arms above your head as you inhale (see Figure 17-2d).**

5. **With your leg still extended in a lunge position, bring your arms back to your sides (see Figure 17-2e).**

6. **Roll your body off the ball by lifting your hips; then place yourself in a kneeling position beside the ball (as Figure 17-2f shows).**

Repeat this sequence two or three times until you feel that your body is completely warmed up and ready to go.

Strong Stretching Poses

The following yoga poses are popular not only for stretching but also for strengthening your arms, chest, glutes, and legs. The shoulders get a workout, too, by becoming the base for the rest of the body.

You can use these stretches as part of your warm-up or cool down and after your regular cardio workout.

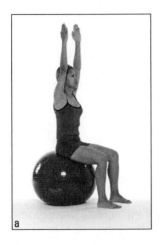

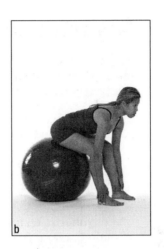

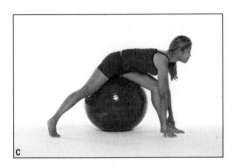

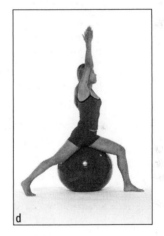

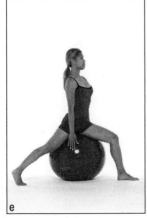

Figure 17-2:
Sun
salutation.

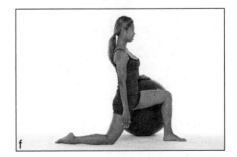

Downward dog

You need to be strong and flexible for this pose. You'll use a lot of upper and lower body strength at the same time.

To do this exercise, follow these steps:

1. **Kneel behind the ball and line your hands up directly beneath your shoulders, placing your hands on the floor on either side of you (as Figure 17-3a shows).**

   Your palms won't be flat on the floor; instead, your fingertips will be touching the floor lightly.

2. **As you exhale, lift your butt toward the ceiling and press your palms into the floor (see Figure 17-3b).**

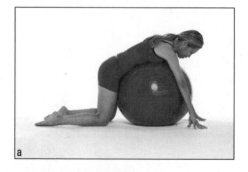

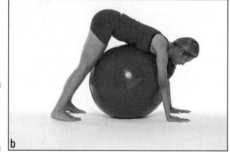

Figure 17-3: Downward dog.

To increase the stretch of this exercise, press your heels down until the balls of your feet are flat and touching the floor.

A couple of do's and don'ts for this exercise:

✔ *Do* keep your breath flowing to release any tension that you may have during this exercise.

✔ *Don't* hyperextend your neck; keep it relaxed and in line with your spine.

Child pose with a rock

Child pose is the position you come into whenever you feel that your body needs a rest. This version has an added rocking movement to help loosen up your neck and shoulders and release any built-up tension.

To do this exercise, follow these easy steps:

1. **Kneel on the floor and drape your body over the ball, letting your head and neck relax to one side (as Figure 17-4a shows).**

2. **Reach your hands forward to the floor in front of the ball and press your butt toward the ceiling (see Figure 17-4b).**

3. **Gently rock forward and back from your hands to your feet. After rocking back and forth a few times, come back to your knees for resting (as Figure 17-4c shows).**

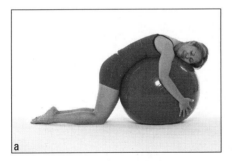
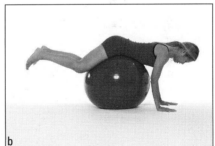

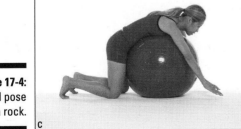

Figure 17-4:
Child pose
with a rock.

Yoga poses for men (and others with tight hamstrings)

Most men have tight hamstrings and are intimidated by yoga because they know they'll eventually have to touch their toes, which is virtually impossible for most men.

But yoga has some really effective and simple poses that anyone with tight hamstrings and even the most manly men can do. Here are a few of those yoga poses that I recommend trying:

The hamstring stretch: In yoga, this stretch is called a *seated forward bend,* and it looks just like the runner's stretch. (A runner's stretch is when you can't do the splits, so you stretch your front leg out and then fold your other leg behind you toward your groin.)

Lower back move: This move is known as the *cat pose.* It really stretches out your lower back in a gentle manner. When you're on your hands and knees, simply arch your back as you lift your face to the ceiling. Then, curl your lower back inward, just as you see a cat do when it wakes up from a really good nap!

The hip opener: You've probably done this exercise before and didn't even know that it was called the *cobbler's pose.* To do this exercise, sit on the floor with the soles of your feet touching. Your inner legs will form the shape of a diamond. Lean forward at your waist to get a more intense stretch. This move stretches out your inner leg, hip, and groin area.

A couple of do's and don'ts for this exercise:

- ✔ *Do* let the ball mold to your body while you relax.
- ✔ *Don't* rock too fast — use a gentle rocking motion instead.

Part IV

Using Exercise Balls in Special Circumstances

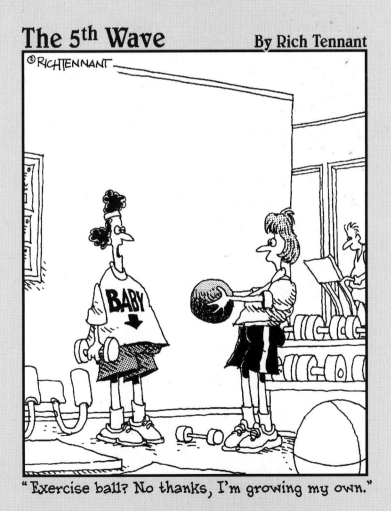

The 5th Wave   By Rich Tennant

©RICHTENNANT

BABY

"Exercise ball? No thanks, I'm growing my own."

In this part . . .

Part IV focuses on special circumstances and, boy, do we have a round-up! I was lucky enough to get a pregnant model (who was ready to deliver in the studio) to show you some great exercises that you can do on the ball throughout your pregnancy. I also lucked out and got the best-looking senior man in town to demonstrate some stretching and strengthening exercises that will help seniors stay fit forever.

Of course, the most fun chapter of all was the kids' chapter. I especially like the "pairs" routines the kids' chapter demonstrates; in this case, I was able to pair up a lovely 7-year-old with a beautiful 11-year-old (who had much longer legs than her partner). Working with the ball can really be for everybody, as you'll soon see!

Chapter 18

Come On, Mama! Pregnancy Workout

In This Chapter

▶ Ball exercises that help you stay comfortable during pregnancy

▶ Using ball exercises to get your body ready for giving birth

▶ Knowing the benefits of working out during pregnancy

▶ Discovering ball exercises that stretch your muscles and build strength

*W*orking out during pregnancy (especially on the ball!) is the best thing you can do for you and your baby. When you use the exercise ball or even sit on one, it elevates the pelvis slightly higher than the knees or brings them just about even. This position instantly creates more space for the baby to move around. Your breathing becomes easier, and your posture also improves. For these reasons, many women find sitting on the ball more comfortable than a chair, especially during their last trimester.

In this chapter, I cover some great exercises on the ball that can make you more comfortable and help you become more flexible. As with any new exercise program, be sure to consult your doctor before starting.

After you give birth and when your doctor gives you the go ahead to work out, the ball can serve as a great tool for strengthening the pelvic floor and pelvic muscles that you haven't used in a while. The exercises in this chapter are also suitable to do during the postpartum period.

Working Out to Ease the Discomfort of Pregnancy

Do you feel like the new package you're carrying around is all in front of you with nothing behind you to help even it out? That's what being pregnant is all about — being a little uncomfortable and a little off-center.

What a rush!

To meet the increased blood supply needed during pregnancy for the placenta and uterus, your circulatory system is working overtime! Dizziness, fatigue, and swelling of the feet and ankles are all signs that everything's pumping along as it should be, despite what a nuisance they may be. If you're dealing with these symptoms, like most pregnant women are, here are a few tips that may help you feel a little better during this unusual but special time:

✔ **Sleep on your left side:** Because sleeping becomes more difficult as the days go by, try sleeping on your left side to allow maximum blood flow to the placenta. You can also try sleeping with a pillow between your legs to balance out the weight of your growing stomach and to alleviate pressure on your back.

✔ **Take it slow:** Because getting up too fast causes sudden shifts of blood away from the brain, always be sure to get up slowly after sitting or lying down for a while. Taking it slow prevents you from becoming dizzy or passing out.

✔ **Drink:** To prevent swelling of the ankles, feet, and hands (otherwise known as *edema*) be sure to drink plenty of water. Sleeping on your left side can also alleviate this problem by enhancing kidney function.

✔ **Walk:** Dangerously high blood pressure (known as *pre-eclampsia*) affects a large percentage of pregnant women, but women who are active during their pregnancy have a reduced risk.

Supporting your body weight and taking the pressure off your back and legs is the best thing you can do to alleviate that uncomfortable feeling. By supporting your lower back in different positions, such as squatting, the ball provides support that would otherwise be placed on the legs — which have way too much strain on them already! The kneeling exercise I cover later in this chapter is especially helpful in supporting the upper body and releasing strain and pressure on the lower back.

To get a complete pregnancy workout that includes cardio, strengthening exercises, and stretching, try pairing the ball workout with swimming. Being in the water leaves you feeling weightless and provides a great way to get the heart pumping and loosen up those muscles.

Why Doesn't My Belly Just Get Big?

Big breasts, a glowing complexion, lots of people holding the door for you . . . who says pregnancy is all that bad? But what about the weight gain? Because you're eating for two, you obviously need a few more calories. And your doctor probably gave you a specific number of pounds that you needed to gain, right? So, where does all this extra weight come from and why doesn't it just go to your belly?

Well, here's the scientific breakdown of your weight gain so you can feel more comfortable as you grow more uncomfortable:

- ✔ **Breast tissue:** This tissue accounts for 2 pounds, and maybe even more for some! (Boy, was I sad to see mine go, although I don't miss the Anna Nicole Smith comparisons! Ha!)

- ✔ **The baby:** Anywhere from 6 to 8 pounds go to the baby, although a lot of woman have preemies who weigh around 5 pounds or babies who weigh well over 10 pounds.

- ✔ **The uterus:** The uterus weighs 2 pounds, and, as you may have heard, it tightens and moves back into place after the baby is born. Your uterus moves back even more quickly when you breast feed. The contractions you feel for a short time after you have the baby also help squeeze out extra fluid and blood from the birth.

- ✔ **The placenta:** The placenta accounts for a 1½ pounds of your baby weight gain. Not bad for being responsible for something as huge as supporting and nourishing your baby while he's in your tummy.

- ✔ **The fluids:** The *amniotic fluid,* which is the fluid your baby is contained in, makes up 2 pounds of your baby weight. When your "water breaks," the amniotic fluid is what's actually "breaking."

- ✔ **The blood volume:** The increase in blood volume (approximately 40 percent) created by your pregnancy to support your growing baby accounts for a whopping 4 pounds. This extra blood is pumping through your veins and pooling in your pelvic area, so keeping yourself moving aids in circulation and keeps the oxygen flowing to support the extra weight and baby within your body.

- ✔ **The fluid retention:** Four pounds of your weight gain is water retention, which your body needs to maintain a balance of nutrients for you and the baby. (Although I can account for about 5 pounds once a month, and so can many of my friends!)

- ✔ **The stored fat:** And last, but not least, the stored fat! The amount of fat that your body stores varies from 4 pounds on up, depending on your diet. This is the one element of your weight gain that you *can* control. Eating better (rather than eating more) while you're pregnant should be your goal.

After giving birth, women lose an average of 22 pounds, so you do the math. Don't forget to take into account how big your baby is and what you weighed before you became pregnant. Having a good body image, taking your pregnancy one day at a time, and savoring and enjoying this special time are important when you're pregnant. And remember: Pregnancy isn't forever!

Reaping the Benefits of Exercise throughout Your Pregnancy

The best time to start exercising is before you become pregnant, but it's never too late to get into a workout program. In addition to the feeling of deep relaxation that exercise gives you, your baby will also benefit. Plus, studies show that working out during pregnancy increases your chances of having a faster and easier delivery and postpartum recovery.

Here are just a few of the benefits you get from exercising during pregnancy:

- Alleviation of back pain, one of the biggest complaints that pregnant women have.
- Increased oxygen to the baby as a result of all the extra breathing that you're doing while exercising.
- Better digestion, which means help with morning sickness.
- Help with labor pains and preparation for delivery. (The stronger your muscles are, the easier your delivery will be because you'll be able to push harder.)

Giving birth has been compared to running a marathon, and that comparison is true — I know from experience! Being in great shape during your pregnancy helps ensure a healthier pregnancy and a faster recovery.

Warming up and cooling down for two

Before you begin working out on the ball, I suggest walking first for 15 to 20 minutes in a shaded area (so you don't get overheated). If the weather is just too hot outside, walk inside with the air conditioning on, at your gym, or at an indoor track at a local school.

When you complete your workout, take a few moments to cool down by "walking it out" at a slow pace for five minutes. When you finish walking it out, take a few moments to slowly inhale and exhale with your arms over your head. This breathing exercise helps you breathe easier and increases the oxygen flow to your baby.

Warming up and cooling down properly is especially important during pregnancy to help your circulation flow freely throughout your body to you and the baby as you begin working out and return to your heart when you're finished.

Great Stretching Exercises for Pregnancy

Stretching releases many of the tensions that you have within your body from a growing girth and an overloaded back. Stretching before a workout is important for everyone, but it's especially important for pregnant women, not only to ease them into movement (which is no easy feat), but also to help keep the blood circulating and the oxygen flowing to the baby. Doing exercises that stretch out or round your back ease discomfort and help your muscles relax. The back roll-up exercise in this chapter and the chest and back stretch are two excellent ways to release built-up tension and discomfort from carrying around your extra weight.

Because of all the extra blood and fluids that your body is producing to support your growing baby, you may feel a buildup of pressure and a pulling sensation in your abdomen. Leg cramps (which I had *really* bad), are also another painful side effect of pregnancy that you can alleviate by stretching your legs and feet first thing in the morning and before you go to bed at night. Doing ankle circles in a chair or at your desk can also help, and even rocking in a rocking chair can relieve leg cramps.

The resting on the ball stretch in this chapter is especially helpful during labor because it can help turn the baby from the *posterior position* (sunny side up) to the correct *anterior position* (when the baby faces down). Believe me, this information is helpful and will definitely come in handy later. Unfortunately, I didn't know that my baby was supposed to be facing downward until the medical team was trying to turn my baby during labor.

Resting on the ball, bouncing on the ball gently, or doing the perineum stretch I include in this chapter can ease your pain immensely *during* labor by alleviating the back pain that comes from the baby pressing on your spine. The motion and movement of using the ball during labor also helps take your mind off the pain.

Perineum stretch

When I was in my last trimester, my doctor told me to get an exercise ball and start sitting on it to stretch out my *perineum*. First of all, I wasn't really sure *what* my perineum was and, second of all, I certainly didn't know *where* it was. Of course, now I know — it's the muscle and tissue that needs to stretch out and be flexible during birth, and doctors may need to cut it in the case of an episiotomy. In other words, the perineum is a place only the ball can support and come in contact with because it's the tissue and muscle that lies between your tushy and your vagina. The following exercise works that hard-to-reach area that comes into play during delivery.

To do this exercise, follow these steps:

1. **Sit up straight on the ball with your feet firmly planted on the ground (see Figure 18-1a).**

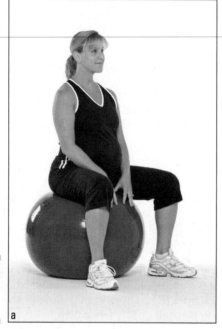 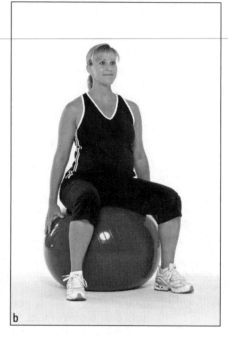

Figure 18-1:
Perineum stretch.

a
b

2. **Place your hands on either side of you so that they're touching the ball (shown in Figure 18-1b).**

3. **Use your pelvis to slowly rotate the ball in a very small clockwise circle.**

4. **Reverse direction and slowly rotate the pelvis counterclockwise.**

Complete ten rotations in each direction and continue the exercise as long as it's comfortable.

A couple of do's and don'ts for this exercise:

✔ *Do* make sure you keep your feet flat on the floor at all times.

✔ *Don't* let your back slouch; keep it straight.

Resting on the ball

Resting on the ball helps many women during labor. By resting your shoulders and chest on the ball, you help alleviate back pain and can help move the baby into a better position for delivery. Because getting comfortable is so difficult to accomplish as your belly gets bigger and bigger, this position is great for alleviating back pain and relieving tension, even if you're not yet near delivery.

To do this exercise, follow these steps:

1. **Kneel on a mat or pillow with the ball in front of you.**

2. **With arms folded, rest your upper body (chest and shoulders) on the ball (see Figure 18-2).**

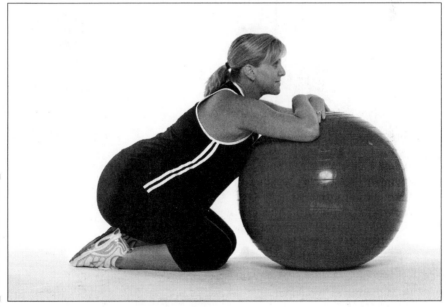

Figure 18-2:
Resting on the ball is a great way to alleviate back pain during labor.

Rest as long as it feels good to you.

A few do's and don'ts for this exercise:

✔ *Do* place a pillow under your butt to make this position more comfortable.

✔ *Do* place the ball against the wall for added support.

✔ *Don't* hyperextend your neck. Keep it relaxed by resting it on your arms.

Chest and back stretch

As you probably know, the number-one complaint among pregnant women is back pain! This comfortable stretch can help release the back and the chest muscles at the same time.

To do this exercise, follow these easy steps:

1. **Sit tall on the ball with your feet hip-width apart.**

2. **Raise your arms out to the side to shoulder height.**

   Your palms should be facing forward.

3. **Stretch your arms behind you as you roll the ball back slightly (see Figure 18-3).**

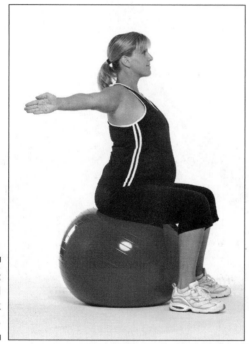

Figure 18-3:
Chest and
back
stretch.

4. **Stretch the chest open by arching your spine gently.**

5. **To reverse this stretch, bring your arms to the front and clasp them in front of your chest, rounding your spine and neck.**

A few do's and don'ts to keep in mind:

- ✔ *Do* breathe through this exercise to increase the stretch.
- ✔ *Do* keep your feet flat on the floor throughout the exercise.
- ✔ *Don't* rush through this stretch. Take your time to relax and rejuvenate for you and the baby.

Back roll-up

The back roll-up helps loosen the upper back muscles. I always like to end my workouts by rolling up the body one vertebra at a time. It feels so good!

To do this exercise, follow these steps:

1. **Sit on the ball with your hands on your thighs.**

2. **Keeping your back straight, lean forward from the hips and hold for a moment (as Figure 18-4a shows).**

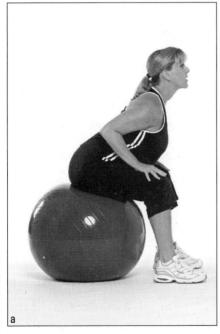
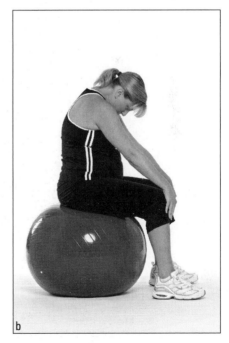

Figure 18-4:
Back
roll-up.

Avoiding overstretching during pregnancy

One of the ways the body naturally gears up for childbirth is to release a chemical called elastin. *Elastin* loosens up all the joints, tendons, and muscles in the body. If you suddenly feel you have the ability to kick your leg above your head like a Rockette, try to resist and stay in the range that was most comfortable to you before you became pregnant.

---

3. **Release your neck and start rolling up one vertebra at a time (see Figure 18-4b).**

4. **Finish the movement by rolling your shoulders back and down.**

Here are some do's and don't for this exercise:

✔ *Do* make sure to roll up slowly — one vertebra at a time.

✔ *Don't* tense up the shoulders. Keep them relaxed and pressed down during this exercise.

Balancing on an exercise ball can be tricky for anyone, especially when you're pregnant. Pressing the ball against an unmovable object, such as the couch or the wall, keeps it from moving around and helps you focus on your workout.

Keeping Up in Arms

One of the biggest benefits to working the arms and upper body before and during pregnancy is the strength that you'll be able to draw upon after you have your tiny new baby. A new baby comes with lots of new stuff to carry around, such as a stroller, car seat, infant carrier, and so on — not to mention the baby, who only gets bigger and heavier with time. And believe me, they can all get pretty heavy after a few trips in and out of the car.

Seated triceps press

On women, flabby triceps are sometimes referred to as "teacher's arms" because, as you probably remember, of the way the skin hung down loosely when your teacher used to write on the chalkboard. Uughh! (Most of the people in my family are teachers, so hopefully they're not reading this.

And if they are, I certainly don't mean any of you!) To prevent teacher's arms, try the following exercises with 3- to 5-pound weights or, if desired, no weights at all.

To do this exercise, follow these steps:

1. **Sit up straight on the ball and firmly plant your feet on the ground.**

2. **Hold weights in both hands behind your head (as Figure 18-5a shows).**

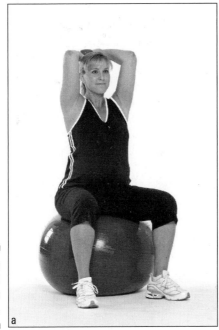 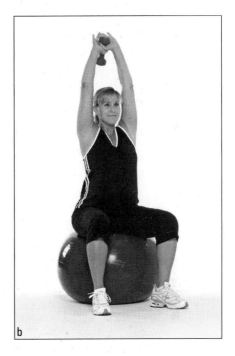

Figure 18-5: Seated triceps press.

3. **Straightening your elbows, press the weights toward the ceiling (see Figure 18-5b).**

4. **Lower the weights behind your head by bending your elbows.**

Complete two sets of ten repetitions.

A couple of do's and don'ts for this exercise:

✔ *Do* keep your elbows close to your forehead.

✔ *Don't* forget to press the elbows straight and to hold that position for a moment when they're pressed above your head.

Wall push-up

The wall push-up tones the entire upper body, including the chest, upper back, shoulders, and arms. This exercise is a modified version of the plank push-up on the ball, and it places less stress on the lower back for pregnant women.

To do this exercise, follow these steps:

1. **Hold the ball at chest height, and press the ball into the wall.**

   Your arms are fully extended, as if you were holding the ball in place.

2. **Bending your elbows out to your sides, slowly press your chest in toward the wall (see Figure 18-6).**

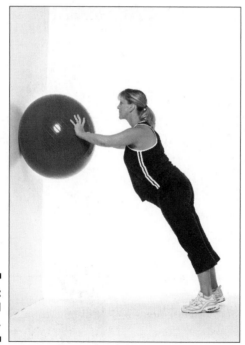

Figure 18-6:
A wall push-up.

3. **Straightening your arms slowly, press back away from the wall.**

Complete two sets of ten repetitions.

A couple of do's and don'ts for this exercise:

    ✔ *Do* move closer to the wall to make this exercise less challenging.

    ✔ *Don't* tilt your pelvis; keep it straight and square to the wall.

Maintaining a Strong Lower Body

The following exercise helps you maintain muscle tone in your lower body while you're pregnant. As you become bigger and heavier, you need to keep your legs strong for carrying around the extra weight. Nothing works better for that than a good old-fashioned squat!

Pelvic rotation

The pelvic rotation works great for alleviating pressure and strengthening your legs while keeping your back and pelvis mobile. The size and weight of your pregnant belly may get in the way as you move your hips around, so try making small circles at first.

To do this exercise, follow these steps:

1. **Sit tall on the ball with your feet shoulder-width apart. Your hands lightly touch the ball on either side of your body (see Figure 18-7a).**

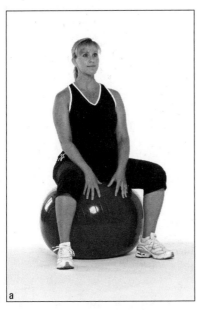 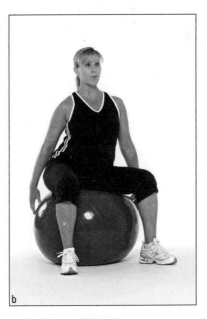

Figure 18-7:
Pelvic
rotation.

2. **Using your pelvis, rotate the ball slowly by pressing down into it. Keep your arms out to your sides for balance (as Figure 18-7b shows).**

   Be sure that your feet remain on the floor at all times, otherwise you can lose your balance and fall off the ball.

3. **Circle your pelvis to the right first and then back to the left in a clockwise fashion.**

4. **End each repetition in neutral spine (that is, sitting tall on the ball without arching your back or tilting your pelvis forward).**

Complete five repetitions to each side.

A few do's and don'ts for this exercise:

 ✔ *Do* sit tall on the ball with a straight back.

 ✔ *Do* use small circles to accommodate your belly.

 ✔ *Don't* forget to exhale as you circle your pelvis.

Wall squats

Nothing's better than a good old-fashioned squat to keep the lower half strong and toned. Using the wall for extra support also gives your back the break it needs during pregnancy.

To do this exercise, follow these steps:

1. **With your feet hip-distance apart, place the ball behind your back and against the wall.**

Snacking is good and alleviates heartburn

Having a snack or something light before you work out is always a good idea. Snacking not only helps you maintain your energy level, but it also keeps you from feeling nauseated. Of course, you don't want to eat a three-course meal but, because you won't be lying on the ball with a pregnant tummy, you won't have to worry about acid reflux or heartburn!

Yes, heartburn, — a BIG problem for pregnant women. And it's another good reason to grab a calcium-rich snack like yogurt. Because the baby is growing so quickly and taking up almost all the room you have left in your tummy, everything is being pushed up, and that doesn't feel good. A small piece of cheese or a glass of milk can relieve your heartburn and give you the boost of energy that you need. Now that's good news!

2. **Place your feet a short distance in front of your torso.**

3. **Press the ball into the small of your back, and start bending your knees as if you were going to sit in a chair (see Figure 18-8).**

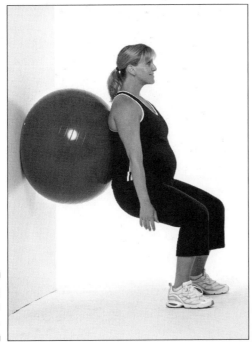

Figure 18-8:
Squats
with a ball.

Make sure that as you bend, your knees don't go any lower than a 90-degree angle.

4. **Hold this squatting position for a count of three, and then slowly come back up to standing.**

Complete five repetitions.

A couple of do's and don'ts for this exercise:

✔ *Do* keep your toes pointing forward.

✔ *Don't* let your knees move beyond your toes.

Chapter 19

Senior Citizens Get on the Ball

. . . .

In This Chapter

▶ Knowing senior fitness and safety guidelines

▶ The ball's benefits: Staying in shape and remaining coordinated later in life

▶ Relieving arthritis pain using strength training and ball exercises

▶ Keeping your lower body strong and flexible

▶ Working and stretching your upper body

. . . .

*A*s people age, coordination and balance begin diminishing, so using the exercise ball to work out makes a lot of sense. First of all, the ball is cheaper than going to a gym and, secondly, playing around with a ball brings out the kid in all of us!

The ball provides an unstable base, which can intimidate some people, but you can do the exercises in this chapter by placing the ball against a heavy coffee table, couch, or wall for added support. By doing so, the ball can roll in only one direction — away from you. As always, consulting with your doctor before you begin any new exercise program is always a good idea.

Why Use an Exercise Ball?

By the year 2020, one out of every four people will be 65 years of age and older. Seniors are, by far, the fastest-growing segment of our population. Because taking care of yourself has never been easier or gotten as much attention as it has been getting right now, there's never been a better time to be a senior! Investing time and money in taking care of your teeth, hair, skin, and so on is undoubtedly important, but just how much you get outdoors to walk and move your body through exercise can determine how active and healthy a lifestyle you can have in your latter years. It's up to you to make small changes in your lifestyle now that will provide you with greater benefits as you age.

So here are a few benefits of working out on the ball that can help you stay in shape for yourself, your grandchildren, your love of gardening, or whatever it is that makes you feel great!

Working out on the ball

✓ **Improves balance and coordination:** Working out on the ball promotes balance and builds leg strength, which can prevent falling — the most common injury among seniors.

✓ **Strengthens your abdominal muscles, which support your lower back muscles:** When you sit on the ball, you engage your core muscles, making them stronger. And strong core muscles provide the support you need for a stronger back.

✓ **Improves flexibility in your hips and pelvis:** Because the muscles in your hips, known as the *hip flexors,* are responsible for the stability of your lower back, keeping mobility in your hips is important as you age. When you sit on the ball, your knees are slightly higher than your hips, which elevates your pelvis and, as a result, helps stretch out your hips.

✓ **Helps maintain mobility in your joints to prevent stiffness:** When the muscles around your joints in your shoulders and knees become stiff, all your movements and simple tasks become more difficult to do. Using ball exercises to maintain your mobility is easier because the ball's shape allows for a wider range of movements than dumbbells or other fitness equipment do.

✓ **Prevents muscle weakness in your legs:** When you don't exercise your muscles, they become weak, which can lead to a loss of control with your movements. Keeping your muscles strong to support your body weight is essential to preventing falls, such as when you're climbing the stairs or stepping down a front porch. By sitting on the ball and lifting your legs one by one, you strengthen your knees and legs at the same time.

✓ **Helps defy gravity:** As you age and your spine compresses from sitting for long periods of time, stretching your spine over the exercise ball counteracts the compression and helps strengthen and elongate your back.

✓ **Provides a workout that you can adjust to your own pace:** Just sitting on the ball engages all your body's core muscles, which provides many benefits, such as postural alignment and the strengthening of your lower back. You can use the ball to replace your chair from time to time or with weights and other accessories (as I show you in Chapter 16), making it one of the most adaptable and easy-to-transport pieces of fitness equipment around today.

Safety Guidelines for Seniors

Do you know the guidelines for senior exercise and how much exercise is recommended? Well, in this section, I tell you just what seniors need to do to ensure safe workouts. I also provide a couple of tips that seniors can do to make working out on the ball safer and less intimidating.

Treating your body kindly

According to the American College of Sports Medicine, seniors should do moderate workouts for 30 to 60 minutes at least twice a week on non-consecutive days — that is, having at least one full day of rest between sessions.

These twice-weekly workouts should consist of exercises that target all your major muscle groups. Seniors should do 10 to 15 repetitions of each exercise using a *moderate level of intensity,* which means 70 percent of the amount of weight you can lift in a single effort. Making a 70 percent effort in your workout should feel challenging but not exhausting to your muscles or require labored breathing. In other words, exercising shouldn't be painful in any way.

The prescribed strength-training routine has safe and effective results when seniors begin it gradually, and increase the number of repetitions over time as they get stronger. Of course, for seniors who are severely out of shape, the "less is more" approach is always better because you can strain muscles and injure yourself by overdoing it. Because seniors are more prone to health concerns when working out, begin gradually using small movements with whatever exercise you choose to do and stop immediately if you feel fatigued or short of breath.

Like with any new form of exercise, consult your doctor before you begin a workout program. Seniors with certain conditions, such as diabetes and coronary heart disease, may have to take a *Graded Exercise Test* (GXT) in which they get on a stationary bicycle or treadmill while their physician monitors their blood pressure and heart rate.

Using a special kind of exercise ball

If the round ball intimidates you or conjures up dodge ball nightmares from your youth, you can use the *Physio roll,* which is an exercise ball shaped like a peanut that's designed for people who need a sturdier base. Because of its

Relieving arthritis pain

Arthritis is the inflammation of a joint (or joints) accompanied by swelling and pain, which affects the spinal column, hips, ankles, and knee joints. It currently affects more than 40 million people and, within a year, more than a million more people will have it. Strength training alleviates arthritis symptoms and slows the aging process by building stronger muscles, bones, and connective tissue.

The American Heart Association recommends that for muscular strength and endurance, sedentary adults use strength training at least twice per week. Although aerobic exercise is great for improving your overall cardiovascular system, it doesn't prevent your body from losing muscle tissue. To maintain muscle mass during seniorhood and to gain relief from arthritis pain, you must perform exercises with weights throughout the later years of your life.

In addition, hip flexors, knees, and ankle joints can become stiff from being sedentary or leading an inactive lifestyle. Using the exercise ball can relieve this stiffness by promoting greater flexibility and mobility in your joints and throughout your entire body.

oval shape, the Physio roll can roll in only one direction and is less likely to slip out from under you when you're working out or sitting on it. You can adapt many ball exercises to the Physio roll and, in my opinion, it's a great choice for many seniors to help build their confidence.

Picking a partner

Using the buddy system when you exercise can help motivate you and keep you safe at the same time. As you get older, losing your balance and your confidence when trying new things is easier to do. Having a workout partner can help you gain back your confidence and boost your self-esteem by having someone else to share in your enthusiasm about your new workout experience and help you avoid injury by having someone else around. And did I mention that exercising is just a *lot* more fun when you do it in pairs? It's much easier to get motivated to go the gym or simply leave the house and take a walk if you know someone is waiting and depending on you.

Working Your Lower Body

When you get out of bed in the morning, does your back feel a lot stiffer than it used to? Maybe you're starting to realize that all those daily tasks like bending over to feed the dog, picking up the newspaper, or taking out the garbage are starting to catch up with you.

To maintain flexibility in your spine, you need to exercise and stretch out your lower back muscles. And what's the biggest benefit to having strong lower back muscles? Being less prone to injury. Now that's good news for anyone. Plus, strong abdominal muscles mean stronger back muscles because these muscle groups work together to form the core of the body. The following exercises are good for both muscle groups.

Abdominal strengthener

The abdominal strengthener is a good exercise to strengthen the abdominal muscles and to help improve posture.

To do this exercise, follow these steps:

1. **Sit tall with a straight spine on the ball and feet hip-width part (see Figure 19-1a).**

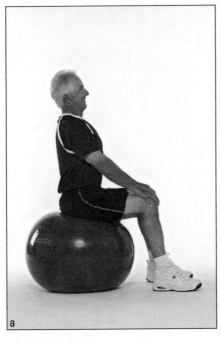 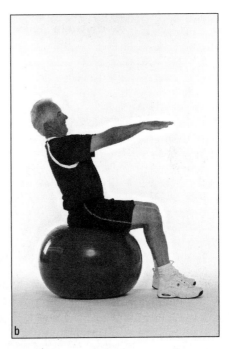

Figure 19-1: Abdominal strengthener.

2. **Hold your arms straight out in front of you to stabilize the body.**

3. **Tilt the pelvis forward slightly and lean back on the ball until you feel your abdominal muscles tighten (see Figure 19-1b).**

4. **Hold pose for the count of three and then return to an upright seated position.**

Repeat five times.

A couple of do's and don'ts for this exercise:

- ✔ *Do* exhale as you lean backward on the ball.
- ✔ *Don't* lean too far backward; stop as soon as you feel your stomach muscles tighten.

Pelvic tilts

Pelvic tilts help keep the upper leg (hips and buttocks) loose and flexible.

To work the pelvis, butt, or gluteal muscles, follow these steps:

1. **Sit tall on the ball with your arms touching the sides of the ball (as shown in Figure 19-2a).**

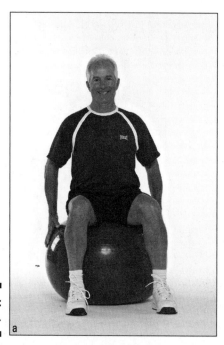
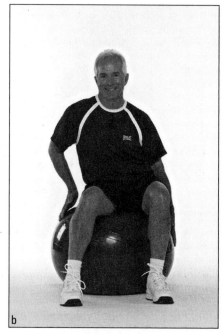

Figure 19-2: Pelvic tilts.

2. **As you tighten the stomach muscles or abdominals, gently push or tilt the pelvis to one side and hold (see Figure 19-2b).**

3. **After holding a few seconds, return to starting position and repeat tilt on opposite side.**

Alternate sides, doing a set of five tilts for each.

A couple of do's and don'ts for this exercise:

✔ *Do* keep your back long and tall during this exercise.

✔ *Don't* lift your feet; keep them firmly planted on the ground.

Leg lifts

Leg lifts improve your balance as well as build strong legs. If you have a two-story house and need to walk up and down the stairs, this exercise really helps strengthen the quadriceps (front muscles of the legs) and the hamstrings (back muscles of the legs).

To do this exercise, follow these steps:

1. **Sit up straight on the ball with your hands touching the sides.**

2. **As you tighten the stomach muscles, lift one leg slowly off the floor and straighten the knee (see Figure 19-3).**

3. **Release the stomach muscles and lower the leg back to the floor. Repeat the exercise on the other leg.**

Complete two sets of ten lifts for each side.

Here are some do's and don'ts for this exercise:

✔ *Do* straighten your knee as much as possible.

✔ *Do* keep the ball still during this exercise.

✔ *Don't* lift the leg any higher than your hip.

Hip strengtheners

As people grow older, the hips become tight and can affect the lower back by throwing everything out of whack. Working the hip flexors help keep mobility in the hips.

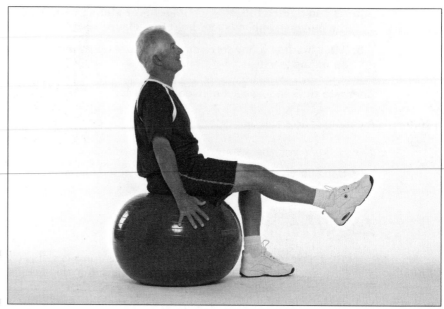

Figure 19-3: Leg lifts.

To do this exercise, follow these steps:

1. **Sit tall on the ball with your feet flat on the floor and shoulder width-apart. Have your hands touching either side of the ball (as Figure 19-4a shows).**

2. **Bend one knee, slowly lifting one leg toward your chest (see Figure 19-4b).**

3. **After holding the pose for a few seconds, return your leg to the starting position and repeat the movement on the other side.**

Here are some do's and don'ts for this exercise:

✔ *Do* keep the ball stable during this exercise.

✔ *Don't* slouch! Keep your back straight and lifted.

Reaching for It

If you have grandchildren, you do a lot of reaching, especially when you pick up stuff off the floor! Because you have to do so much reaching and extending, you need to stay flexible and loose. Plus, fighting off arthritis is one of the greatest benefits of staying flexible, so go for it!

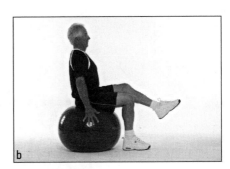

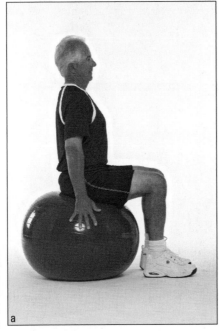

Figure 19-4:
Hip
strengthener.

Side reach

The side reach exercise helps prevent stiffness. Doing this exercise upon waking up is good to loosen up the body and prepare for the day.

To do this exercise, follow these steps:

1. **Sit on the ball with your feet shoulder-width apart. Raise your right arm as you tighten your abdominal muscles.**

2. **With your left arm, slowly bend to one side, reaching down the side of the ball (see Figure 19-5).**

3. **Hold the pose for a few seconds and then return to the starting position. Repeat on the other side.**

Complete five to ten stretches on each side.

Here are some do's and don'ts for this exercise:

  ✔ *Do* keep your stomach muscles tight to support your weight.

  ✔ *Don't* hold your breath as you reach to the side.

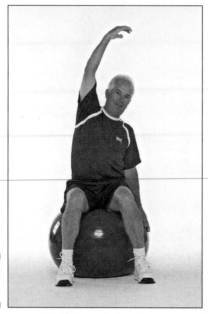

Figure 19-5:
Side reach.

Shoulder roll

As I mention in the earlier sidebar called "Relieving arthritis pain," staying arthritis-free or keeping your joints from getting stiff is a big concern as people get older. The shoulders can become very tight and tension can build up. The shoulder roll exercise helps keep the muscles from getting stiff and keeps them nice and loose around the shoulder joint.

To do this exercise, follow these steps:

1. **Kneel on an exercise mat or some kind of cushion, draping your arm over the ball (as Figure 19-6a shows).**

Exhale with effort

I always have a hard time remembering when I'm supposed to inhale and when I'm supposed to exhale during an exercise. Breathing at the right point in an exercise makes such a difference because it helps increase your stretch and release stress. Next time you're about to begin working out, remember to inhale as you begin and exhale with effort. Proper breathing makes things so much easier!

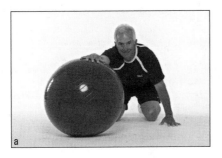

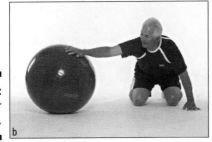

Figure 19-6:
Shoulder
roll.

2. **Use your shoulder to slowly roll the ball out to your side as if you were drawing a half circle outside your body. End your movement when the ball is even with your feet (see Figure 19-6b).**

   Be sure to use only your shoulder to move the ball and keep your body facing forward.

3. **Slowly roll the ball back up the side of your body toward the top of your head.**

Complete five rolls on each side of the body.

A couple of do's and don'ts for this exercise:

✔ *Do* face forward during this exercise.

✔ *Don't* lean to the side or bend at the hips.

You can do this exercise in a seated position on the floor if kneeling is too painful. Simply move the ball from the front of the body to the rear of the body while you're seated on the floor.

The drape

This exercise is a favorite of many chiropractors because it naturally stretches your back muscles by using the gravity of your own weight. Adding a gentle rock to the drape is soothing and mild at the same time.

To do this exercise, follow these steps:

1. **Kneel behind the ball and rest your arms at your sides.**

2. **Drape your body over the ball face down. Rest your fingertips and your feet on the floor for support (as Figure 19-7 shows).**

   Let your head and neck relax toward the floor.

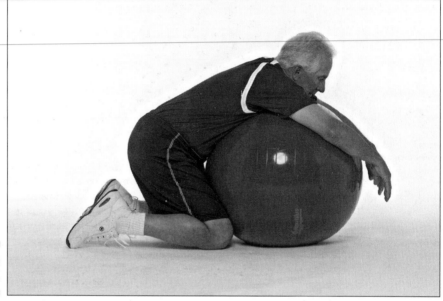

Figure 19-7:
The drape.

3. **Rock gently back and forth, releasing your back of any built-up tension or tight muscles.**

4. **Come back into starting position and rest on your knees before repeating the stretch.**

Repeat three to five times.

A few do's and don'ts for this exercise:

- ✔ *Do* let your body relax toward the floor during this exercise.

- ✔ *Don't* forget to breathe, which allows your back muscles to release farther toward the floor.

- ✔ *Don't* forget to let your head and neck hang down in a relaxed position.

Chapter 20

Every Kid Loves a Ball

. . . .

In This Chapter

▶ Tips for working out with your kids

▶ Finding the right ball size for kids

▶ Bouncing and rolling exercises kids love

▶ Pairing up for ball exercises

. . . .

Seeing kids really enjoying a physical activity that benefits them in so many different ways is wonderful and fun. My 2-year-old and I have done all the exercises in this chapter together, and she just loves them! Every day she asks me to put her "on the ball" and, to my amazement, she has memorized the sequence of the floor exercises!

I designed the last two exercises in this chapter to do with a partner, which makes them even more fun and challenging for the whole family. Feel free to pair up brothers with sisters, cousins with aunts or uncles, and even parents to have a great time and to loosen up a little bit in the process.

For a final stretch, try the drape and the backbend stretch, which I include in Chapter 10. With smaller kids who are around 2 to 3 years old (like mine), you can actually place them on the ball for both of these exercises and gently roll them back and forth. The exercises are so soothing and relaxing that you'll have to hide the ball because I guarantee your kids will want to do them over and over!

For parents, I assure you that this workout is anything but a waste of time for you. Many of the exercises I include in this chapter for your kids I also use for adult workouts in other sections of this book. With a little modification (that is, speeding things up a bit), you can get a great workout and have so much more fun doing it alongside your kids. And maybe your kids will even challenge you to try something new and fun!

Workin' Out and Having a Ball

Most kids like to really go for it when they first try something new — like running head first into a pile of leaves or throwing themselves down a slip and slide at break-neck speed. You have to admire that kind of enthusiasm.

In the spirit of making things go as smoothly as possible the first time out, here are a few important workout tips that kids need to know before they get started:

✔ Make sure that your kids follow the instructions in this chapter thoroughly.

✔ Make sure they don't hold their breath during the exercises. Holding their breath won't help them perform the exercises any better and will only leave their little lungs short of oxygen!

✔ Have them perform each exercise without straining or injuring themselves.

✔ Make sure they use a smooth surface for the ball workout to avoid puncturing the ball.

✔ Be sure they use a slow and steady motion when doing each exercise until they become pros at it — which, for kids, means at least once or twice.

✔ If they feel dizzy or short of breath during any of the exercises, have them stop and take a break.

✔ Make sure your kids use the ball only as this chapter demonstrates. In other words, keep an eye out in case one of your little ones just can't resist the urge to try standing on the ball or hurling it at her baby brother.

Finding Just the Right Ball Size for You and Your Little One

Most kids need to use the smallest ball because ball sizes go according to height. For instance, the 45 centimeter ball measures 22 to 24 inches in diameter, depending on how much air you use to inflate your ball, and is recommended for ages 3 and up. My daughter loves this ball, and it's great for balancing, bouncing, and exercising. The 24 inch ball can hold up to 180 pounds, so most adults can use it, too.

The recommended ball height is one that allows your legs to make a 90-degree angle (right angle) at your knees when you're sitting on the ball with both feet flat on the ground. If you're still not sure that your ball is the correct height, filling the ball slightly bigger so your hips are higher than your knees is better than filling it too little so that your knees are higher than your hips, because this places unneeded strain on your knees.

Filling your ball to the brim with air should be reserved for people who are experienced working out on the ball. If you fill your ball with too much air, staying on it is difficult because it's so taut. You need to fill it only to the point that it feels comfortable or has a little give when you sit on it.

Bouncing and Rolling Workout

I designed the following workout with kids who haven't actually sat on a ball before in mind. The heel touches and side steps are good exercises to start off with to encourage good balance and coordination. The marching and bouncing are good cardio exercises that get the blood flowing and the heart pumping — plus, they're just plain old fun to do.

I designed the two exercises at the end of this workout — the hamstring stretches and ball pushes — for you to do in pairs; these exercises are meant to add a bit of variety. Just be sure that you have plenty of space to roll around — and don't forget to play nice!

Heel touches

The object of this exercise is to keep the ball still as you reach out with your leg and touch alternating heels to the floor. Believe me, doing this exercise isn't as easy as it looks!

To do this exercise, follow these steps:

1. **Sit tall on the ball with your feet shoulder-width apart and your hands at your sides (as Figure 20-1a shows).**

   Your hands will lightly touch the ball for support.

2. **As you extend your right leg in front of you, reach out with your right heel (see Figure 20-1b).**

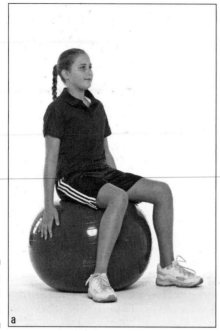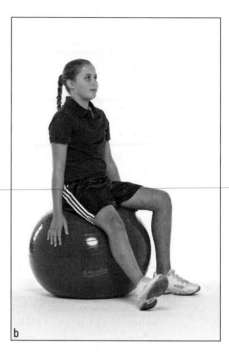

3. **Return your right heel back to starting position before extending your left leg and heel to the opposite side**.

Alternate heel touches for two sets of 10 to 15 repetitions.

When you feel comfortable and balanced on the ball, try speeding up the movement.

Some do's and don'ts for this exercise:

✔ *Do* keep your back straight as you reach your leg out and place your heel on the ground in front of you.

✔ *Don't* let both your feet leave the ground at the same time. Always keep one foot on the floor.

Marching

Marching is always fun for kids, especially when done on the ball. The key to this exercise is to raise the knees as high as possible without losing your balance and falling backward off the ball.

To make moving to the beat as you march more fun, try turning on some music with a fast-pace tempo or drum rhythm.

To do this exercise, follow these steps:

1. **Sit tall on the ball with your feet shoulder-width apart and your hands at your sides.**

2. **As you tighten your stomach muscles for support, lift your left leg as high as possible (as Figure 20-2a shows).**

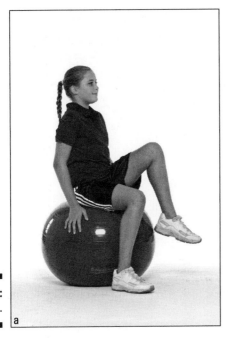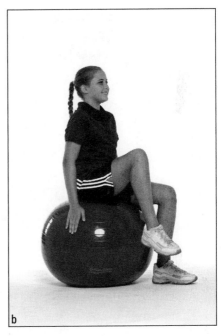

Figure 20-2:
Marching.

a   b

3. **Alternate lifting both legs in a marching fashion (see Figure 20-2b).**

Continue marching for a few minutes until you feel your hips are warmed up and ready to go.

A few do's and don'ts for this exercise:

✔ *Do* keep your knees pointing straight out in front, not out to the side, during this exercise.

✔ *Do* keep your hands on the ball at either side of you for support.

✔ *Don't* let the ball move; keep it as still as possible.

Side steps

By reaching with alternate legs while on the ball, the side step simultaneously opens up the pelvis and works the legs.

You really have to be careful to maintain your balance while extending each leg to the side. To keep from falling off the ball, sit up straight and maintain perfect posture for this exercise.

To do this exercise, follow these steps:

1. **Sit tall on the ball and place your hands on either side of you.**

2. **Extend your right leg out and to the side, straightening your right knee (as Figure 20-3a shows).**

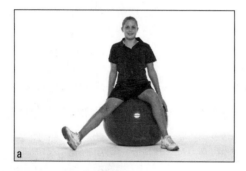

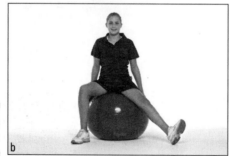

Figure 20-3:
Side steps.

3. **Slowly bring in your right leg and extend your left leg out to the opposite side (see Figure 20-3b).**

Complete 15 repetitions.

A few do's and don'ts for this exercise:

- ✔ *Do* keep your hands behind your body and on either side of you for support.

- ✔ *Do* straighten your leg as far as possible as you extend it to the side.

- ✔ *Don't* lean forward on the ball as you step out with your alternating leg. Keep your back straight and lifted.

Bouncing

I love balls that have handles on them so you can leapfrog around the room. Because the exercise ball doesn't have handles to grasp onto, you have to use your center of gravity and your hands to guide you as you do small bounces up and back down onto the ball.

Try placing the ball against a wall or a heavy object, like a couch, as you do this exercise. Doing so keeps the ball from moving so that when you jump up and come back down, the ball will be right where you left it!

To do this exercise, follow these steps:

1. **Sit tall on the ball with both hands on either side of your body.**

2. **Using your legs, jump up straightening your knees (as Figure 20-4a shows).**

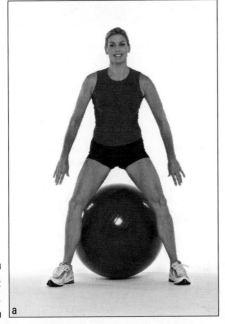
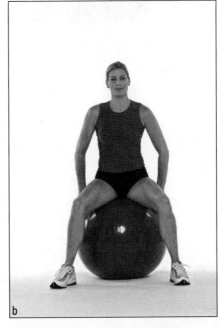

Figure 20-4: Bouncing.

a

b

3. **Return to the starting position, being sure to replace your hands on either side of your body and back onto the ball for support (see Figure 20-4b).**

Complete a series of 10 to 15 bounces before you rest and begin another set.

A couple of do's and don'ts for this exercise:

✔ *Do* use your leg and butt muscles to lift you off the ball rather than using your hands.

✔ *Don't* jump too high off the ball. Remember that you're bouncing, not jumping.

Family Style: Pairing Up for Ball Exercises

The next two exercises are extra fun because you do them in pairs! Use your sister, brother, mom, or dad to push the ball back and forth. You can even make a game out of the hamstring stretch exercise by having all your family members sit with their legs outstretched and push the ball back and forth in a circle. Kind of like playing Twister, but you're sitting!

Doubles: Ball pushes

Doing ball pushes is a great way to release tightness that you may have built up in your back. This exercise is also great for helping your kids develop teamwork skills because they'll have to guide their partner through a series of pushes and pulls.

To do this exercise, follow these steps:

1. **Lie on your back with your knees bent into your chest. Using both you and your partner's feet, hold the ball up between you (as Figure 20-5a shows).**

   The ball will be exactly in the middle of both people.

2. **Without touching the floor, extend your legs and slowly move the ball back and forth between you and your partner (see Figure 20-5b).**

Complete 10 to 15 repetitions.

A couple of do's and don'ts for this exercise:

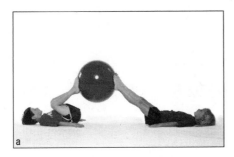

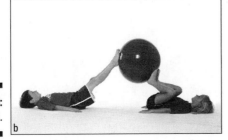

Figure 20-5:
Ball pushes.

✔ *Do* use the abdominal muscles to support the movement of the ball.

✔ *Don't* let your back arch away from the floor; keep your back pressed down and use your feet to guide the ball.

Doubles: Hamstring stretches

This exercise stretches your legs and helps build coordination.

Pairing up different age groups for this exercise is fun. Just make sure that smaller kids are big enough to reach the ball when they extend their legs out and to the side.

To do this exercise, follow these steps:

1. **Place the ball between you and your partner and sit on the floor with your legs stretched out and toes lightly touching (as Figure 20-6a shows).**

   Your hands will be on top of the ball.

2. **Tightening your stomach muscles and sitting up straight, push the ball forward to your partner and hold for a few seconds (see Figure 20-6b).**

3. **Sit up in the starting position before you reverse the movement.**

   Push the ball back and forth, holding for a few seconds in between the 10 to 15 repetitions.

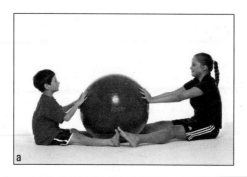

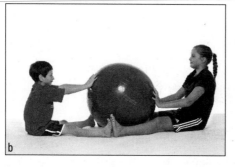

Figure 20-6: Hamstring stretches.

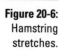

A few do's and don'ts for this exercise:

- ✔ *Do* use an exercise mat if the ball starts to roll too much.
- ✔ *Do* stretch forward or extend from your hips when you push the ball to your partner.
- ✔ *Don't* let your neck fall forward. Keep your head lifted and in line with your spine.

Family health

According to the American Heart Association, overweight children who don't exercise are likely to become overweight adults who don't exercise. These kids are at risk for developing type-II diabetes during childhood as well as other problems and diseases that can plague them well into adulthood. Depression, poor body image, low self-esteem, and obesity are just a few. Fortunately, the same goes for children reared in a healthy environment — they're likely to become healthy grown-ups.

Letting kids just plop down in front of the TV after school is easy to do. Raising lazy and overweight kids are two major concerns of parenting these days. In fact, the American Heart Association reports that 10 percent of children are overweight and spend an average of 17 hours a week watching TV.

Providing a healthy environment means providing one that's full of fun activities where kids can thrive. And the fitness industry is offering just that kind of environment with family exercise classes. These classes are becoming more and more popular because studies have shown that kids' levels of physical fitness go down significantly between the ages of 12 and 18 and adolescent weight gain goes up. That's why parents are helping to motivate their kids by joining them in a fitness class that is designed for the entire family. Swimming classes, yoga, aerobics, circuit training, and karate are just a few of the types of classes being offered for the family at local recreational facilities.

Even if your family can't participate in family exercise classes, you still have plenty of options that can keep your family healthy. Take a walk in the park with the family dog, play volleyball at the beach, fly a kite, or go for a nightly jog together. These activities are all great examples of what you can do as a family for the sake of exercising. Not only are you and your kids toning your bodies, you're also fine-tuning your family relationships.

Part V
The Part of Tens

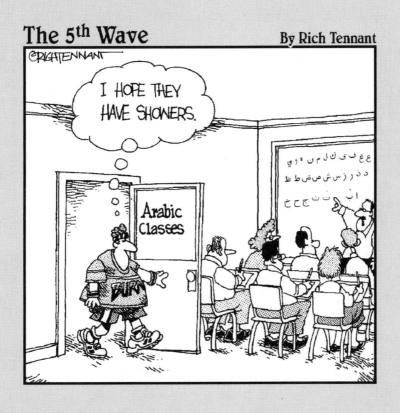

In this part . . .

In every *For Dummies* book, you find top-ten lists at the very end. In this part, I tell you the ten changes you can expect to see in your body, more about who can use the ball, ten ways to complement your workout, and what you can't do with the ball!

It's a fun part, so read on.

Chapter 21

Ten Changes You Can Expect to See in Your Body

In This Chapter

▶ Finding out what a difference working out with the ball makes

▶ Discovering all the benefits of using the ball

*T*his chapter tells you about all the exciting changes you can expect to see in your body from using the ball. Besides developing good overall muscle tone for your entire body, the ball provides numerous other benefits, ranging from rehabilitating back, hip, and knee injuries to improving your core stability. (And don't forget that the ball delivers great posture and improves muscle imbalances, too.) The ball also increases your circulation by delivering a low-impact workout that revs up your cardiovascular system.

If you happen to be pregnant or a senior citizen, I highly recommend taking a look at Chapter 18, where I list the benefits of using the ball during pregnancy, or Chapter 19, where I cover the benefits for seniors. For now, though, read on to find ten great changes that everyone can expect to see from using the ball.

Improved Posture

For many years, experts believed that the best way to protect your back and keep it injury-free was to have a "flat" back. Nowadays, doctors have found that maintaining the slight natural curve in your spine is even better. When your spine is in this natural alignment, a person has good posture.

When you use the ball, you have to sit up straight (as your mother probably told you time after time) to keep the ball steady and to maintain your back's natural curve. The ball provides better posture, giving you a more graceful appearance, by improving your balance as you try to hold yourself steady on the ball and maintain your core control and keep from falling off. Training on the ball is one way to work the hard-to-reach group of stabilizer muscles.

Just by sitting on the ball, you're able to activate the stabilizer muscles and not only improve your posture but also get more in touch with your center of gravity. After only a few workouts, you'll appear taller and thinner from your improved posture and be able to maintain perfect posture longer throughout the day. Plus, you'll get a lot of compliments because everyone notices good posture!

Increased Flexibility

One of the ball's greatest strengths is its ability to give you a good stretch. The reason is because the ball's shape allows you to drape your body over it, stretch backward on it, and get into positions you probably never thought were possible.

Your hamstrings, hips, and back are the tightest areas in your body. Because many people choose exercises that are mostly for building muscle mass, they forget to stretch out after their workout, which leads to tight, sore muscles and inflexibility. Men are particularly susceptible to this problem because they have more muscle mass than women. Still, plenty of women have flexibility problems, too.

The good news is that training on the ball improves flexibility. You can use the ball to do back stretches and loosen up tight hamstrings using a series of easy stretches that show great results in just a few sessions; Chapter 14 offers a great stretching workout.

After you use the ball just a few times, you'll feel more flexibility in your back and abdominal region, which makes you stand taller and look thinner! Both women and men . . . I guarantee it!

Tighter Buns

Because you're using major muscle groups — like your glutes — just to stay seated on the ball, you'll see a difference in your butt right away. You can find some killer exercises in Chapter 9 (called "Booty Patrol") that'll make a difference in your derriere and give you that much-desired poochy look in no time.

Training on the ball develops good muscle tone for the tushy because you recruit these larger muscle groups in your body for balancing the ball. You will need to squeeze your glutes to stay seated on the ball and engage your abdominals to keep you lifted and steady. So while you're training one muscle group, you use the other for balancing, which provides good overall toning as well.

For example, while you're lying with your back on the floor and your lower legs on the ball, you need to press down and into the ball by tightening your glutes and using the weight of gravity of your legs. Defying gravity through certain exercises on the ball helps you defy gravity throughout life so you maintain a nice rear view!

Stronger Abs

Yes, you can get a six-pack by using the ball (something you can't achieve with yoga or Pilates). Your core, which used to be called your midsection, is made up of the deep abdominal and back muscles that work as stabilizers for the entire body. These muscles are the "deep" muscles because, although you can't see them, they're responsible for maintaining the core stability in your body.

Working these inner muscles, or your core, is extremely hard to do. But you can work them using the ball because it allows you to train your deeper abdominal muscles even though other pieces of fitness equipment don't. By pulling in your abdominal muscles and tightening your *pelvic floor* (the group of muscles at the end of your pelvis), you're able to hold the ball steady and develop the tight, toned tummy you've always wanted.

Less Lower Back Pain

Working out on the ball is great for people with back problems because it supports their lower backs as they exercise and stretch. And that's exactly why physical therapists and chiropractors started using the ball.

Using the floor to push against or lie on doesn't have the versatile quality that the spherical shape of the ball provides. While you're stretching over the ball, you benefit from the gravitational pull downward that allows your body to open up in a very non-invasive manner. A feeling of weightlessness comes over you when you're working with the ball that's hard to achieve with other equipment or exercise. And the ball's pliable surface feels soft to the touch and, at the same time, is strong enough to support all your body weight.

To feel how great the ball is for your lower back, check out the drape and other stretching exercises in Chapter 14, which you can use as a series of strengthening exercises for your entire back area.

No wonder physical therapists and chiropractors understand the many benefits of the exercise ball and prescribe using them regularly not only for rehabilitation but also just to help patients get back in touch with their bodies.

Enhanced Balance and Coordination

By balancing on the ball, you teach yourself better coordination and make yourself more graceful in the process. As you're in motion on the ball, you'll need increased balance to have full control over the ball and all your movements. So when you're rolling one way, you need to use the resistance of your own body weight to steady the ball as you stop and roll in the other direction. You'll see the difference in your balance and coordination in no time — and probably be walking like a ballerina after a few short workouts!

Improved Range of Motion

When you use the ball and lift weights, you gain a fuller range of motion because the ball's shape doesn't keep you from doing a full arm circle (as you would on a weight bench). For this reason, the ball has become a great tool for physical therapists. Being able to strengthen your grip with the natural shape of the ball or to move it around for various seated and lying positions gives you the ability to train in all directions.

You can even get a cardiovascular workout by using different choreography with the ball; for instance, you can lift it over your head, bounce it in front of you, or sit and bounce on it! The ball is truly an amazing, unlimited tool for increasing and improving your full range of motion.

Easier Maintaining of Neutral Spine

One of the principle factors in using the ball is maintaining a *neutral spine.* The ultimate goal in trying to achieve a neutral spine is to keep the natural curve in your spine without overcorrecting it. In other words, to stabilize your back, your hipbones and your pelvis need to be on the same plane.

Being in neutral spine is really an active position where the lower abdominal and pelvic stabilizer muscles are engaged to create a "girdle" of sorts for the entire body. If you were standing, your pelvis would be pointed straight down to the floor or dropping straight down. The proper way to describe a neutral spine while a person is standing up tall is neither arched nor tilted forward.

When you work with the ball, you need to sit tall and maintain a neutral position in your spine to keep the ball from rolling away. You also need to control your body positioning to maintain the correct alignment needed for you to stay seated on the ball.

When you are lying on the floor or with your tummy on the ball in the prone position, you'll have the most control of the ball by keeping it as close to your core as possible to decrease the challenge and maintain your balance. As you become stronger and more confident with your ball workout, you can increase the difficulty by moving the ball further away from your body's core.

After a few short sessions, you'll be able to maintain the proper alignment needed to exercise on the ball. If you don't sit up straight in neutral spine, you'll get automatic feedback when you fall off the ball!

Muscle Balance

When one muscle group is stronger than its opposing muscle group (like the triceps and biceps for example), this is a *muscle imbalance*. Because muscles need to work together to perform common tasks such as lifting and pushing, it's important that both of the muscle groups involved in the movement be equally strong.

Many times people train the front muscles in their bodies but neglect the back muscles. This situation creates muscle imbalances that can be difficult to correct. The ball offers a solution to muscle imbalances by providing a way to strengthen posterior and anterior muscle groups (front and back) while supporting the lower back.

In addition, you can easily modify ball exercises to target your particular muscle imbalances. When you identify a muscle imbalance, you can work to even it out by strengthening the imbalance through exercises that use the ball as a base of support for resistance, or you can add a few pieces of equipment to it.

For example, if you wanted to strengthen your hamstrings, you'd lie on the floor with your lower legs on the ball and lift your hips as you steady the ball and press your legs and glutes down into the ball. To modify the movement and make it less difficult, you would move the ball closer to your torso, or core, of the body. As you progress, you would move the ball away from your body's core toward your lower legs and feet to increase the level of difficulty.

To avoid muscle imbalances and to look and feel good whether you're coming or going, you need to train your buttocks, back, hamstrings, chest, and upper body.

Increased Circulation

Want to get that glow or be heart healthy? Performing exercises on the ball not only increases your circulation, but it also burns fat! Because you're using so many different large muscle groups, which elevates your heart rate, using the ball as a training tool helps keep your heart rate elevated through-out your workout. (Just make sure you're working at just a steady regular pace.)

You can do all kinds of exercises on the ball to increase your circulation and enhance your workout. The cardio workout in Chapter 5 is challenging and will get your heart rate up in no time. I suggest always adding five to ten min-utes of walking before and after your ball workout to properly warm up and cool down your body. Warming up helps prevent injuries and prepares your muscles and body for the exercises and movements that are about to come. Cooling down helps the blood to return back to your heart and allows your breathing and body temperature to return to normal.

I also suggest adding some form of resistance to the ball (as Chapter 16 shows) to burn more calories and to add a new dimension to your workout. If you really want to test your endurance and build muscle mass at the same time, the weight-training routine in Chapter 13 provides you with a workout that will do just that.

The total-body workout in Chapter 11 is also an excellent way to stretch, tone, build, elongate, and keep you fit for a long time to come.

Improved circulation helps you develop a strong cardiovascular system, which helps prevent chronic illnesses and the possibility of injuries later on in life. The results of improved circulation can be a smaller risk for heart dis-ease, an increased energy level, and a better sex drive! That sounds like a good reason to get the heart pumping, now doesn't it?

Chapter 22

Ten Groups That Can Use the Ball

In This Chapter

▶ Finding out who can benefit from using the ball

▶ Getting familiar with different groups that need to exercise

*E*veryone from elite athletes to new moms are using exercise balls not only to make ordinary exercises more challenging but also to increase circulation and flexibility. Traditional exercises like simple abdominal crunches become more effective when you do them on the ball because you're engaging your core muscles that don't get used when you're lying on the floor or on a workout bench. Plus, you get results twice as fast because exercises on the ball improve your muscle strength and endurance by engaging the small stabilizing muscles that are difficult to train with other forms of exercise. And another plus of sitting on the unstable surface of the ball is that you enhance your balance and coordination as you improve your posture.

So whether you're a beginner or a senior, the following list tells you specifically why training on the ball helps improve your level of fitness and why it's the new way to go when you need to get a great workout.

Athletes

Elite athletes are probably the group most responsible for bringing the ball to the public's eye. The media paid a lot of attention to athletes when they started using them to train for sports-specific skills, such as balance. You have to admit, seeing Shaquille O'Neil on a ball (a large ball, of course) in the news was a pretty funny sight. But Shaq says it's a great tool for teaching coordination and other skills that basketball players need to use on and off the court. You may have seen the ball make an appearance at the Olympics, too. Swimmers use the ball to loosen up their joints and to prevent lower back strain caused by weakened muscles.

Athletes use exercise balls to help them get an edge over the competition and to stay injury-free. Here are some other reasons athletes train using the ball:

- ✔ To improve sports-specific skills
- ✔ To increase flexibility
- ✔ To increase endurance
- ✔ To develop balance
- ✔ To aid in training of hand-eye coordination
- ✔ To strengthen connective tissue throughout the body to enable lateral movements that many sports require
- ✔ To warm up their body and increase their core temperature before competing

Beginners

Beginners are people who've never been on an exercise ball before or are new to exercising. Whatever your definition of a beginner is, you'll benefit from using a modified base of support to train with (otherwise known as the ball) because you're better able to gain perfect balance and coordination than if you use the floor or a weight bench.

In addition, you can see changes more quickly on a beginner's body because she's probably using her *core,* or internal muscles, for the first time in her life.

The following list tells you why training on the ball is so beneficial for beginners. Beginners can use the ball to

- ✔ Acquire stability.
- ✔ Develop balance.
- ✔ Increase flexibility in their muscles.
- ✔ Enhance future training.
- ✔ Get a low-intensity cardiovascular workout by maintaining an elevated heart rate.

Bodybuilders

Bodybuilders traditionally work out on a weight bench. But when bodybuilders use the ball as their base instead of a bench, the core muscles become engaged and provide a more intense workout (see Chapter 13). Keeping your body steady while sitting on the ball and lifting heavy weights is quite challenging and should only be done by experienced weight lifters.

Here are some ways that using the ball as a base helps train bodybuilders in a more challenging way:

- Alters the base of support

- Provides added resistance

- Improves muscle imbalances

- Trains and defines core muscles

- Teaches hand-eye coordination

- Develops good balance

 Chapter 13 is a weight-training chapter that shows different techniques you can use with weights when you're using the ball as your base of support instead of a weight-training bench.

Hyperactive Children

Children love the ball! For this reason, doctors incorporate exercise balls into therapy to help hyperactive children maintain a stronger focus and learn how to slow down and take a break.

Children also respond to the playful, fun element of using an exercise ball, but most importantly, they're learning skills that help them become more coordinated. The ball is soothing and strengthening, which makes it a wonderful tool for helping children overcome hyperactivity. Through the use of specific exercises and games that are provided by your doctor or teacher, hyperactive children can learn to have fun while developing important skills that will help them improve their condition. (Don't forget to ask your doctor about exercises you can do at home to help your child.)

Here are other benefits that kids get from having a ball. Children with Attention Deficit Disorder (ADD) and hyperactive children use balls

- To improve focus and concentration.

- To learn and develop coordination.

- To define spatial problems.

- To improve overall fitness level.

Even if your children aren't hyperactive, try getting them to do the ball workout in Chapter 20, which I designed *especially* for kids.

New Moms

What better way for new moms to tighten and tone their slackened abdominal muscles than working out on the exercise ball? The ball is a great training device for new mommies because it's an easy in-home workout.

New moms can also use the exercise ball soon after their delivery as a cushion to relieve stress on the area where painful episiotomy stitches are. Additionally, the ball eases the stress and strain that labor placed on the lower back.

Here's a list of ways that new moms can use the ball to gain relief and how they can incorporate them into their workout programs:

- To tighten and tone abdominal muscles after having a baby

- To strengthen the pelvic floor after birth

- As a base to perform Kegel exercises to help them gain back bladder control

- To increase circulation

- To provide a low-intensity cardiovascular workout

- To ease the pain of episiotomies by providing a soft, cushiony base

Pilates Students

Because keeping the ball from moving around (or rolling around) is difficult, the ball is a great tool for teaching challenging exercises that require small movements and strength, like the Pilates method. In addition, the unstable base of the ball complements many of the Pilates-based exercises otherwise known as *mat exercises*.

Combining the ball with Pilates exercises also gives Pilates students better posture and improves their balance when they try to remain steady on the ball. And because the exercise ball is light and portable, it's easier to transport and more versatile than other pieces of Pilates equipment, which are cumbersome and may take up a lot of space (like the Pilates reformer, for example).

So combining all the principles and benefits of these two powerhouse forms of exercises seems perfect. Like anything that's paired as a team, the results can be twice as good and twice as rewarding!

Here are some more ways in which Pilates students benefit greatly from using the ball:

- ✔ To assist in training core strength, or the deeper abdominal muscles, that other pieces of fitness equipment don't target
- ✔ To teach techniques that many Pilates exercises emphasize
- ✔ To provide a base for non-impact movements
- ✔ To increase the balance challenge of Pilates' mat exercises
- ✔ To add variety to their workout

Chapter 12 introduces you to doing Pilates on the ball and starts you out with some basic exercises.

Pregnant Women

Pregnant women can benefit greatly from using the ball because it provides a comfortable place to sit, and it supports their growing tummies (which gets harder and harder to do later during pregnancy).

Another name for the exercise ball is the *birthing ball*. Women sometimes use the birthing ball during labor because it helps alleviate pain by providing a supportive base that encourages movement for pregnant women. Because movement is soothing for a woman going through labor, the slight rocking motion can also help turn a baby in the mother's womb into the correct position in the birthing canal.

The following list provides a few more ways in which pregnant women use the ball for support and comfort:

- ✔ To stay flexible
- ✔ To stay comfortable as their tummies grow
- ✔ To alleviate back pain from the added pressure of carrying around a baby
- ✔ To ease the pain of labor with light bouncing
- ✔ To help turn the baby into the correct position in the birthing canal

TIP

Head to Chapter 18 for a great ball workout that's specially designed for pregnant women.

Rehabilitative Patients

Physical therapists first used the ball to alleviate their patients' injuries. The exercise ball provides a way to support the lower back without causing pain, so it's the perfect training tool for someone who's just undergone back surgery.

People who are limited in their range of motion because of surgery or who are recuperating from shoulder and neck injuries need to increase their ability to move in all directions to avoid stiff joints and muscles. The ball provides a full range of motion to help these patients recover fully. In addition, the ball helps patients develop good muscle tone throughout their bodies by recruiting major muscle groups to provide overall toning.

Here are a few more reasons patients use the ball to help them recuperate more quickly from surgery or injuries:

- ✔ To relieve back pain
- ✔ To strengthen hip and knee joints during post-surgery treatment
- ✔ To improve muscle imbalances
- ✔ To correct postural alignment

Seniors

As people get older, their coordination and balance begin to diminish. You can use the exercise ball to maintain these vital abilities. Because the ball provides an unstable base and may intimidate seniors, placing it against a heavy coffee table, couch, or wall for added support keeps the ball from rolling around.

As people age, the disc spaces in the lower back narrow due to over-use and gravity. The result is a stiff, tight lower back. You need to move these muscles and stretch them (in other words, exercise), which is just as important, if not more so, than it was when you were younger.

The exercise ball is a perfect training tool to revitalize your body and help keep it strong and injury-free. Doing simple stretching exercises on the ball provides flexibility, which helps seniors maintain their daily lifestyles and activities.

Following are some more ways that seniors can use the ball to stay perfectly fit for a long time to come:

✔ To improve their circulation

✔ To improve their posture

✔ To stretch and bend (which helps prevent falls)

✔ To increase mobility

✔ To decrease stiffness in their joints

✔ To relieve tightness in the muscles

✔ To maintain coordination for a lifetime

Chapter 19 offers a great workout tailored to the needs of senior citizens.

Yoga Students

Yoga is hugely popular these days, and rightfully so. It's a challenging undertaking that requires great strength, especially in your upper body. Most people who take a yoga class come out of it with a real appreciation and new respect for those who practice yoga regularly.

Because yoga can be extremely demanding and because it requires great flexibility, combining it with the ball makes it more accessible and easier for beginners. For experienced yoga students, the ball offers a fresh and new opportunity to take their training to a higher level by using a new approach.

Here are just a few ways the ball enhances the practice of yoga. Yoga students use them as

✔ An added base of support for moving through postures.

✔ An aid to make yoga accessible to more people who are less flexible.

✔ A base that provides progression to roll through different challenging poses and positions.

✔ A way to increase or decrease the level of training in various poses.

If the idea of practicing yoga on the ball intrigues you, check out Chapter 17.

Chapter 23

Ten Activities That Complement Your Ball Workout

. . . .

In This Chapter

▶ Discovering the right forms of exercise to use with the ball

▶ Knowing what you can do to get a better workout

. . . .

*T*he ball itself provides an intense workout. When you combine the ball with some form of cardio or strength training, you can get faster results.

Depending on the type of ball workout you choose to do, this chapter offers a way to mix and match exercise programs that will take you to a higher level of fitness.

Jumping Rope

Remember when you used to jump rope as a kid? Well, jump ropes have made a comeback, and rightfully so. Boxers use them, athletes use them, I love them, and you can use them to warm up and cool down quickly. And if you've tried one recently, you already know they provide a good cardiovascular workout.

In fact, here's a reason why all women should love jump ropes: They're the only device out there that can actually take away that little bit of cellulite on your body. The small jumping movement you use helps speed up your circulation and flush out some cellulite. Jumping rope for as little as five minutes a day is all it takes to keep your butt and legs looking more toned and dimple free.

Jumping rope is a quick and easy way to complement your exercise ball program because it's inexpensive and all you need is five minutes of it before you're ready to get on the ball. After five minutes, your body will be warmed up and ready for anything (and you'll have a nice glow from all that blood pumping through your veins). Jumping rope also creates shapely shoulders and a tone upper body, which makes it a perfect complement for a lower body workout on the ball as shown in Chapter 9.

So jump to it and you'll feel the difference in no time!

Walking

Walking is good for everybody, even when it's cold outside. Plus, everyone can do it and it's free — so no excuses! Adding a walking routine to your ball workout is a good idea because it stretches your legs and gets your body warmed up or cooled down in no time.

To warm up, I suggest starting at a slow pace and gradually increasing to a faster pace. For a cool down, do the opposite: Start with a quick pace and gradually decrease to a slower pace.

Whatever ball routine you decide to do, adding a brisk 15- to 20-minute walk to it will keep you flexible and your heart healthy. Walking also helps strengthen the muscles in your lower body (legs and butt), which helps you stay fit and trim because bigger muscles burn more fat.

Spinning Class

Spinning is what you do on special spinning bikes, which look like stationary bikes, at the gym. You can usually see 15 or so people in a spinning class racing like mad dogs as the teacher sits in front of the class instructing them.

Taking a spinning class is a good way to burn calories. Because the wheels on the bikes weigh around 40 pounds, you can burn up to 500 calories! As well, because the wheels weigh 40-plus pounds, you're doing a weight-bearing exercise that builds muscle and strength in your entire lower body and burns fat for the entire hour. Now that's a good class.

If you took one or two spinning classes a week along with working out on the ball the same amount of times per week, you would look and feel like an athlete in no time. I'm sure of it!

Finding a Partner

Getting motivated to exercise is sometimes hard, isn't it? Well, an easy solution to this problem is to draft a friend to be your exercise buddy. Walking with someone in your neighborhood or training with someone at the gym makes exercising easier and more fun. Plus, you can motivate each other when one of you doesn't feel like training, taking a class, or whatever activity you both choose to do.

Plus, using the buddy system is safer when you go for walks and when you use weights. Having a friend there can help prevent falls and injuries that you may otherwise get when you work out by yourself.

Be sure to check out the partner exercises on the ball in Chapter 20 in this book. You'll find a few great exercises for enhancing lower body strength and coordination.

Kickboxing

You've heard of Tae Bo, right? Kickboxing classes are good for toning and strengthening your lower body, and they provide a good cardiovascular workout.

Most kickboxing classes use the exercise ball as a training device, too. After all that punching and kicking, the instructor usually has you work your abs and strengthen your core on the ball. Now, that's what I call a one-two punch!

After you finish a kickboxing class, a great way to wind down and increase your flexibility is with the yoga on the ball exercises as shown in Chapter 17.

A Workout Video

An exercise video is good for figuring out a new exercise technique in a one-on-one setting, where you don't have to feel embarrassed if you don't get the moves down right away.

Exercise videos are very effective tools that are handy and convenient. You'll never have an excuse not to pop in a video and work out.

There are some very good videos that use the ball to give a killer cardio workout that can compliment any strength training program. If you lift weights two to three times a week, I suggest using a cardio ball video two times a week to give you a full body workout and round it all out.

Martial Arts

Karate, kickboxing, and other martial arts are great training tools for the body and the mind. For that reason, martial arts complement the ball well. Training with martial arts also promotes flexibility, strength, and endurance through calisthenics and kicking exercises that provide a good cardiovascular workout and overall toning of the body. When you use the ball, you need to increase your focus and concentrate so you don't fall off. Martial arts stresses the same kind of mind-body connection that you need to succeed when you're using the ball.

Ballet

If you like ballet, you're probably familiar with the ball because many dancers use them. Ballet classes are good for toning your entire body and creating long, lean legs and arms. Ballet also gives you better balance and coordination, which is useful when working out on the ball.

Ballet can relieve lower back pain by elongating the key muscles that control your pelvis and back area, such as the hamstrings (upper leg muscles that run along the back side of the leg), lumbar muscles (lower back muscles), hip flexors (pelvis or hip muscles), and glutes (butt).

Other benefits of ballet include increasing the core temperature of your body, which enhances flexibility and makes your movements easier to perform throughout the day, and providing a fat-burning workout through a series of dance movements that keep your heart rate elevated.

Stretching

Stretching is a good complement to any kind of workout. If you don't stretch, your body becomes stiff and tight. And your back, well, that's a whole other subject!

Everybody's flexibility differs because each individual's joints are different. Some people can stretch like a rubber band, whereas others have a hard time touching the floor with their hands. Of course, the goal of stretching is to extend your range of motion so that everyday activities are easy and effortless to perform.

Stretching is great for reducing stress because it increases the blood supply to tight, tense muscles. It also promotes better posture by realigning and strengthening the muscles that support coordination and movement.

Most importantly, stretching reduces injuries because it helps you gain control over your body's movements and your range of motion. You can use many different techniques to enhance your stretching; they are listed in Chapter 14.

A good way to add stretching to your workout program is to join a yoga or mat Pilates class. Both classes are equally effective for revving up your circulation and increasing your flexibility.

Rest

Resting is good for your body and your overall health. Resting for 24 to 48 hours between workouts is not only recommended by the Department of Health and Human Services, but it's also needed for the body to recharge itself and replenish your fluids to avoid dehydration or muscle soreness.

If you don't take the time to rest between workouts, you may experience muscle fatigue or muscle burnout and ruin all your hard work by injuring yourself.

Knowing how to maintain balance in your life is just as important as knowing how to maintain balance with your body and health. Next time you feel like you're doing too much in the gym or even around the house, take a few days off, and you'll soon see how much better off you'll be when you're able to lift more weight and run faster.

Chapter 24

Ten Things You Can't (Or at Least Shouldn't) Do with Your Ball

. . . .

In This Chapter

▶ Discovering where you can't take your ball

▶ Knowing what not to attempt on your ball

. . . .

*T*his chapter is kind of like watching one of those crazy shows on TV where they say "don't try this at home because it can be dangerous"! There really are some things you can't do with your ball, although I know some of you have tried! Check out the ten instances in this chapter to see whether you're one of those people who like to do the impossible — or make that the improbable.

Stand On It

Although some bodybuilders and competitions teach techniques for standing on the ball, I beg you not to try it. Standing on the ball isn't safe, and you don't get any major physical benefit from it.

Sit, don't stand. The ball wasn't made for standing for obvious reasons!

Take It Inflated on an Airplane

Okay, this one may sound kooky, but I've seen someone try it. Bringing an inflated ball on a plane isn't recommended and certainly isn't allowed. Simply deflate it and pump it up whenever you get where you're going.

Work Out in an Area That's Too Small

Working out in an area that's too small is a no-no. You can puncture the ball by rolling over something or, worse yet, injure yourself when you whack your head or arm on a coffee table. So make sure you clear enough space before you begin your workout.

Slick It Up with Oil or Other Products

Now, slipping around on the ball may sound like a fun time, but it's not. Don't wear lotions or oils while using the ball. Doing so just adds to the slippery surface, and you could get hurt.

Wear Spiked Shoes While Using the Ball

I cover what to wear in the beginning of this book (see Chapter 4), and I guarantee that spiked shoes aren't on the list. You could puncture the ball and land flat on the floor. Ouch!

Use It in the Water

Some floats look like balls and noodles and all kinds of stuff, so use those in the pool, but don't use your exercise ball in the pool. The ball isn't designed for use in water because it can be harmed by the chlorine and other chemicals, and more importantly, I don't want you to get hurt.

Pump It Too Full of Air

I cover air levels in Chapter 3, but you should know by now not to fill it too full. Just like a bike tire or balloon, an exercise ball can pop if it's over-inflated, and then you'd have to go out and buy another ball. Plus, if the ball's too full, you won't be able to work out on it properly because the ball needs to have a little give to it.

Pop It with a Pin

Well, duh. But along these same lines, don't wear belts or other gadgets that may puncture the ball when you're lying or sitting on it.

Use It Next to a Heater

The ball can overheat, expand, and then pop. If you have a radiator or electric heater nearby, you could melt your ball if it rolls in that direction. Also, keep your ball away from extreme changes in temperature — hot or cold — because it causes the air pressure to build up inside the ball and burst.

Take It in the Snow

Alright, so taking the ball in the snow does sound fun. But like I said before, the ball is susceptible to heat and cold and can burst when it expands, so don't take it outside in the snowy weather or use it on the ice. In addition to damaging the ball, you could damage an arm or an ankle. Ouch!

Index

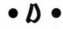

• M •

• N •

NESS, CAREERS & PERSONAL FINANCE

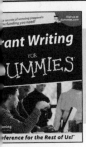

nt Writing

0-7645-5307-0

Home Buying

0-7645-5331-3 *†

Also available:
- Accounting For Dummies †
  0-7645-5314-3
- Business Plans Kit For Dummies †
  0-7645-5365-8
- Cover Letters For Dummies
  0-7645-5224-4
- Frugal Living For Dummies
  0-7645-5403-4
- Leadership For Dummies
  0-7645-5176-0
- Managing For Dummies
  0-7645-1771-6

- Marketing For Dummies
  0-7645-5600-2
- Personal Finance For Dummies *
  0-7645-2590-5
- Project Management For Dummies
  0-7645-5283-X
- Resumes For Dummies †
  0-7645-5471-9
- Selling For Dummies
  0-7645-5363-1
- Small Business Kit For Dummies *†
  0-7645-5093-4

E & BUSINESS COMPUTER BASICS

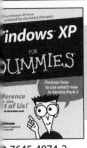

indows XP

0-7645-4074-2

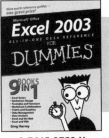

Excel 2003

0-7645-3758-X

Also available:
- ACT! 6 For Dummies
  0-7645-2645-6
- iLife '04 All-in-One Desk Reference
  For Dummies
  0-7645-7347-0
- iPAQ For Dummies
  0-7645-6769-1
- Mac OS X Panther Timesaving
  Techniques For Dummies
  0-7645-5812-9
- Macs For Dummies
  0-7645-5656-8

- Microsoft Money 2004 For Dummies
  0-7645-4195-1
- Office 2003 All-in-One Desk Reference
  For Dummies
  0-7645-3883-7
- Outlook 2003 For Dummies
  0-7645-3759-8
- PCs For Dummies
  0-7645-4074-2
- TiVo For Dummies
  0-7645-6923-6
- Upgrading and Fixing PCs For Dummies
  0-7645-1665-5
- Windows XP Timesaving Techniques
  For Dummies
  0-7645-3748-2

O, HOME, GARDEN, HOBBIES, MUSIC & PETS

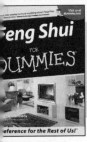

eng Shui

0-7645-5295-3

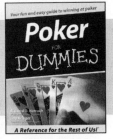

Poker

0-7645-5232-5

Also available:
- Bass Guitar For Dummies
  0-7645-2487-9
- Diabetes Cookbook For Dummies
  0-7645-5230-9
- Gardening For Dummies *
  0-7645-5130-2
- Guitar For Dummies
  0-7645-5106-X
- Holiday Decorating For Dummies
  0-7645-2570-0
- Home Improvement All-in-One
  For Dummies
  0-7645-5680-0

- Knitting For Dummies
  0-7645-5395-X
- Piano For Dummies
  0-7645-5105-1
- Puppies For Dummies
  0-7645-5255-4
- Scrapbooking For Dummies
  0-7645-7208-3
- Senior Dogs For Dummies
  0-7645-5818-8
- Singing For Dummies
  0-7645-2475-5
- 30-Minute Meals For Dummies
  0-7645-2589-1

ERNET & DIGITAL MEDIA

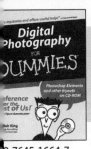

Digital Photography

0-7645-1664-7

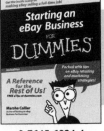

Starting an eBay Business

0-7645-6924-4

Also available:
- 2005 Online Shopping Directory
  For Dummies
  0-7645-7495-7
- CD & DVD Recording For Dummies
  0-7645-5956-7
- eBay For Dummies
  0-7645-5654-1
- Fighting Spam For Dummies
  0-7645-5965-6
- Genealogy Online For Dummies
  0-7645-5964-8
- Google For Dummies
  0-7645-4420-9

- Home Recording For Musicians
  For Dummies
  0-7645-1634-5
- The Internet For Dummies
  0-7645-4173-0
- iPod & iTunes For Dummies
  0-7645-7772-7
- Preventing Identity Theft For Dummies
  0-7645-7336-5
- Pro Tools All-in-One Desk Reference
  For Dummies
  0-7645-5714-9
- Roxio Easy Media Creator For Dummies
  0-7645-7131-1

 WILEY

SPORTS, FITNESS, PARENTING, RELIGION & SPIRITUALITY

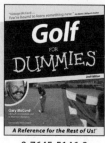

0-7645-5146-9

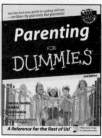

0-7645-5418-2

Also available:

- Adoption For Dummies
  0-7645-5488-3
- Basketball For Dummies
  0-7645-5248-1
- The Bible For Dummies
  0-7645-5296-1
- Buddhism For Dummies
  0-7645-5359-3
- Catholicism For Dummies
  0-7645-5391-7
- Hockey For Dummies
  0-7645-5228-7

- Judaism For Dummies
  0-7645-5299-6
- Martial Arts For Dummies
  0-7645-5358-5
- Pilates For Dummies
  0-7645-5397-6
- Religion For Dummies
  0-7645-5264-3
- Teaching Kids to Read For Dumr
  0-7645-4043-2
- Weight Training For Dummies
  0-7645-5168-X
- Yoga For Dummies
  0-7645-5117-5

TRAVEL

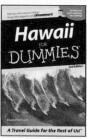

0-7645-5438-7

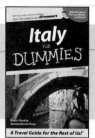

0-7645-5453-0

Also available:

- Alaska For Dummies
  0-7645-1761-9
- Arizona For Dummies
  0-7645-6938-4
- Cancún and the Yucatán For Dummies
  0-7645-2437-2
- Cruise Vacations For Dummies
  0-7645-6941-4
- Europe For Dummies
  0-7645-5456-5
- Ireland For Dummies
  0-7645-5455-7

- Las Vegas For Dummies
  0-7645-5448-4
- London For Dummies
  0-7645-4277-X
- New York City For Dummies
  0-7645-6945-7
- Paris For Dummies
  0-7645-5494-8
- RV Vacations For Dummies
  0-7645-5443-3
- Walt Disney World & Orlando For Du
  0-7645-6943-0

GRAPHICS, DESIGN & WEB DEVELOPMENT

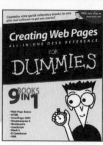

0-7645-4345-8

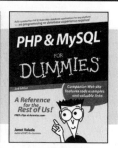

0-7645-5589-8

Also available:

- Adobe Acrobat 6 PDF For Dummies
  0-7645-3760-1
- Building a Web Site For Dummies
  0-7645-7144-3
- Dreamweaver MX 2004 For Dummies
  0-7645-4342-3
- FrontPage 2003 For Dummies
  0-7645-3882-9
- HTML 4 For Dummies
  0-7645-1995-6
- Illustrator CS For Dummies
  0-7645-4084-X

- Macromedia Flash MX 2004 For Du
  0-7645-4358-X
- Photoshop 7 All-in-One Desk
  Reference For Dummies
  0-7645-1667-1
- Photoshop CS Timesaving Techni
  For Dummies
  0-7645-6782-9
- PHP 5 For Dummies
  0-7645-4166-8
- PowerPoint 2003 For Dummies
  0-7645-3908-6
- QuarkXPress 6 For Dummies
  0-7645-2593-X

NETWORKING, SECURITY, PROGRAMMING & DATABASES

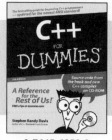

0-7645-6852-3

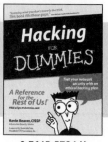

0-7645-5784-X

Also available:

- A+ Certification For Dummies
  0-7645-4187-0
- Access 2003 All-in-One Desk
  Reference For Dummies
  0-7645-3988-4
- Beginning Programming For Dummies
  0-7645-4997-9
- C For Dummies
  0-7645-7068-4
- Firewalls For Dummies
  0-7645-4048-3
- Home Networking For Dummies
  0-7645-42796

- Network Security For Dummies
  0-7645-1679-5
- Networking For Dummies
  0-7645-1677-9
- TCP/IP For Dummies
  0-7645-1760-0
- VBA For Dummies
  0-7645-3989-2
- Wireless All In-One Desk Referen
  For Dummies
  0-7645-7496-5
- Wireless Home Networking For Du
  0-7645-3910-8